THE ONE HOUR TRAINER

90 Day Roadmap To Building A Successful And Profitable Fitness Business That You Love

By: Rahz Slaughter & Greg Kalafatic

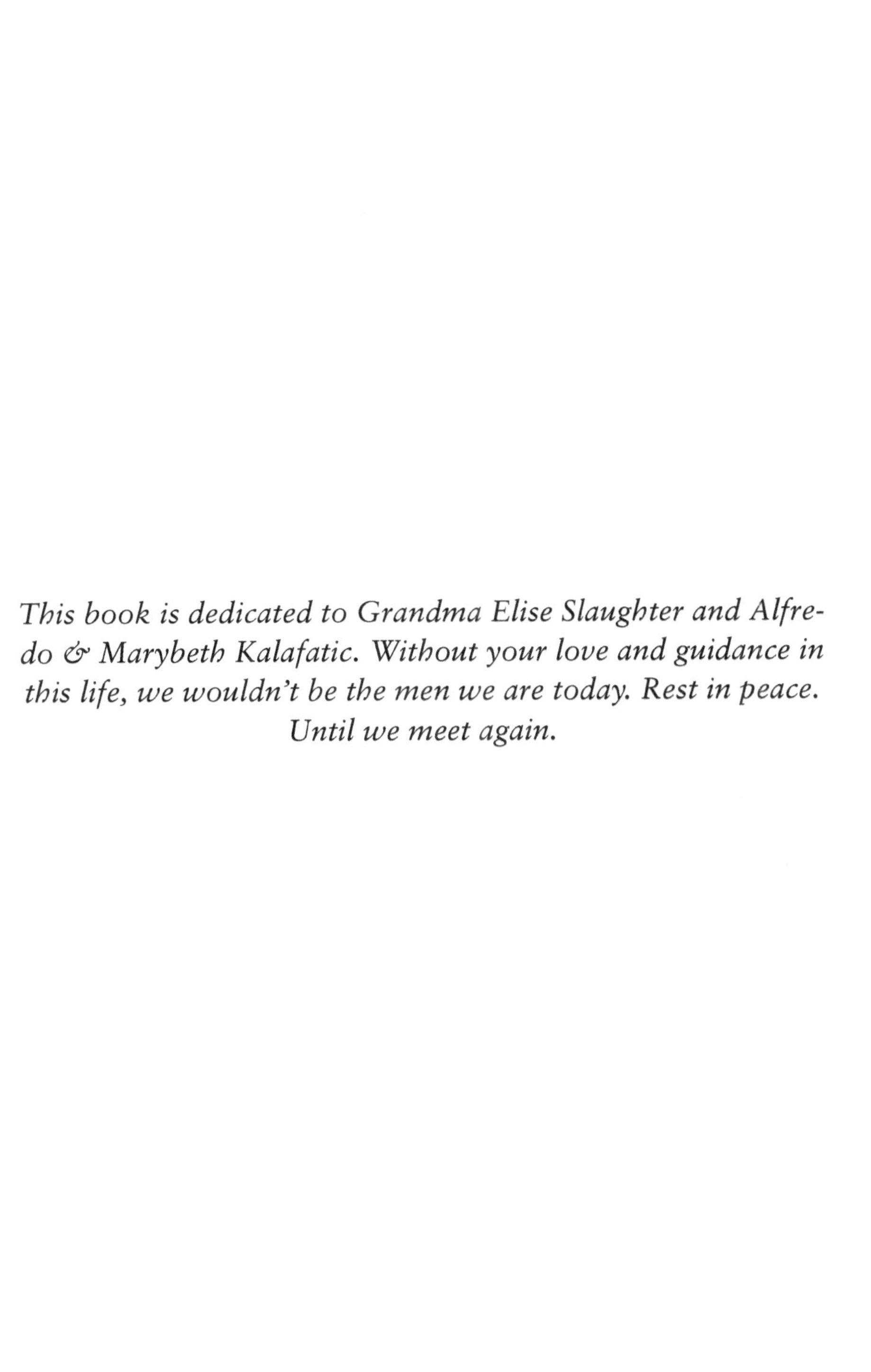

This book is dedicated to Grandma Elise Slaughter and Alfredo & Marybeth Kalafatic. Without your love and guidance in this life, we wouldn't be the men we are today. Rest in peace. Until we meet again.

Contents

PART 2: SELL

Chapter 4 — GENERATE DEMAND

PART 3: SYSTEMIZE

Preface

1 hour.

60 minutes.

3600 seconds.

Have you ever thought what you could do in an hour?

I know you picked up this book and thought 'Hey this must have something to do with that other book, *Four Hour Work-week,* by Tim Ferris.' If you guessed that, you're absolutely right. We wanted to call the book *Four Hour Trainer* but did not want Tim to get mad at us; we actually like his work and what he is teaching people through his whole four-hour brand.

All joking aside, if you've picked this book, there are a few things that I will take a wild guess on. You want more time. I do not know what you want to do with the more time, but nor does it matter. What does matter is you having the choice to decide what to do with your time. For many in the fitness business industry, we, unfortunately, cannot decide what to do with our time. Our businesses dictate what our time looks like. The 5 am training sessions, the 12 pm sweep up of the gym because no one ever comes at that time, then the 5 pm after work mad rush to the gym only to leave the gym late at night and repeat this cycle all over again. How many of you started a fitness business hearing this is the typical lifestyle and thought that it would not go down like that for you? Perhaps you thought I could figure out a way to make it different. You might be one of the few that actually love that work schedule, and if that is you, that is okay too, but let me ask this…

How's your LIFE?

What do you do when you are not at the gym? What is it like to always be working when your friends want to grab dinner, or your family wants you to spend more time together? What is it like when your weekends are tied down for morning and mid-afternoon sessions because the business does not generate enough money for you to be closed during those hours? In this day and age, many fitness professionals leave the profession frankly because they have to sacrifice a life in order to make a living. This is not living. It's surviving. It's what leads to such high turnover in the fitness industry. It's what drives business owners to mistreat their workers because they are overwhelmed with bills and fires to put out and are underwhelmed with the life that they live.

In *One Hour Trainer*, you will get a behind-the-scenes look at two guys who literally started from the bottom. What's the bottom, you ask? Read the introduction; it will reveal what humble beginnings look like for someone looking to build a fitness business. You will get a chance to look in the mirror and see how your current lifestyle is no different than other fitness business owners who all started with the same dream only to experience the same nightmare.

What if I was to tell you that this does not have to be your story and you can actually build your dream business? What if I told you that you can make a great living and actually live, not just survive? What if weekends could be weekends again and evening dinners with those who matter most to you could once again be on the table?

No matter what current challenge you are facing or lifestyle you are living, there is ALWAYS a solution to turn things around. It breaks our heart knowing that something like fitness brought us all so much joy, yet for most, it becomes the biggest frustration.

This book is here to share with you what it takes to not only share the gift of health with the market you serve, but also for you to be the benefactor of building a business that provides a great lifestyle that you actually love.

As you dive into this book, there are certain reactions that you will experience. First will be the up and down nod. The up and down nod will happen when you read an experience that you can relate to. This book is relatable because we were you as you'll read. The next reaction is the SMH (shaking my head). You will shake your head when you read about something that reminds you of a past frustration that you've dealt with or one you are dealing with. The second to last reaction will be the :O, which is an emoji that shows you are shocked. This will happen when you read about the case studies of people who just like you nodded up and down, shook their head, and now are living a lifestyle they dictate and no longer let their business dictate their lifestyle. The last but not least reaction you will have is one of enthusiasm. When you read the principles that are shared in this book, you will realize that there is nothing special about us, but what is special are the strategies that we used and how they can work for EVERYONE who reads this book.

Are you ready to dive into the book? Ready to learn what it takes to build your dream life and dream business where they actually work in sync?

Well then, turn the page and let's get started on this journey together where it all started for us.

INTRODUCTION:

Steve Jobs once said, "You cannot connect the dots looking forward, you can only connect them looking backwards. So you have to trust that the dots will somehow connect in your future." This quote really sums up what every entrepreneur at some point in their journey has felt. We hope that the dots connect in the future and all the hard work and labor was all worthwhile. The book you are holding in your hands today is going to pull back the curtains a bit to show you exactly how those dots connected. Before doing so, we thought it would be important to know the backstory of how this book came to be. Without the history, you won't truly understand the story and see how our story can very well be your story. We'll address how two guys who did not grow up together were able to build a lifestyle fitness business that allows us to essentially run a fitness business instead of a fitness business running us to the ground. Let's start by telling you a little about us and how we connected as there are some important lessons that if missed will derail your plans on building on the information shared later.

Who Is Rahz Slaughter?

You normally do not think about who you are until it's too late, like in your obituary, but in simple terms, I'm a personal trainer, a coach, a stepfather, a husband and a loyal friend. This would be the equivalent of what you see on a sports trading card, but that only includes basic stats without the mention of the stories that help those stats be and the people who were there or not to make it all possible. I am someone who has had a humble beginning because my life started out with a birth defect. Before I was given a name, my first label was given to me. I was born disabled; my right leg was shorter than my left leg. I have no quadriceps or hamstring on my right leg. I was also born with a dislocated hip, which was the first thing that they had to fix when I was born. Talk about a tough beginning.

Have you ever felt like something went wrong from the get-go? Almost like it was not meant to be? What about adding to the equation that my father left my mother and me at the hospital, when he walked away saying, "I don't want a child, and I don't want to be a part of this child's life." So, here's a recap thus far on my first day on earth:

- Disabled

- Dislocated hip

- Dad-less

While my start was filled with difficulties, I thank God that my mother decided to keep me. It most certainly was not easy for her being a 19-year old woman, raising a child without the father present and not having an education. With just a basic GED, she was able to make it through that tough process because of the love and help of my grandmother, our rock when we hit rock bottom.

My grandmother is the most inspirational and motivational woman that I've ever known. She passed a couple years ago, but credit goes to her for the man I am today. The things she taught me, I would use to overcome the challenges that lie ahead of me. For example, when it came to school, I was not a scholar at all. I barely got out of high school. I actually never read a book until I was almost 19-20 years old. I lost my reading virginity to the book "Norton Reader" while in Europe, where I did not have any television and thought about reading short stories for entertainment. That is when I got hooked on reading. Because I was no longer in school, I taught myself how to read. This became my next challenge, as I skipped words while reading, thus giving me no comprehension of what I was reading. Little did I know then, I was dyslexic. All my life, I did not know I had this disability. Even when I was in reading classes, I had no idea.

As you can see by now, being labeled disabled was a theme in my life. No father and a drug-addicted mother, to learning how to read while being dyslexic. The odds were stacked against me, but I did not want those labels to define my story. I didn't want my story to be about the disadvantages life gave me. Instead, I wanted it to be about how I was able to take advantage of the opportunities presented to me. I had a knack for being able to see things differently, which leads me to my journey into the fitness industry.

As if it was yesterday, I can remember where my love for fitness came from. As a kid, I loved working out and doing pushups. I would do pushups with my uncle, and as encouragement, he gave me a quarter. The more and more I did it, the stronger and stronger I became. That's a tip in itself. The more you do it, the better you'll be able to do it. I utilized my strength throughout junior high and high school to avoid getting picked on. I was also a decent athlete, turning myself into an All-American, top-rank wrestler in high school and college.

To think that I was one day told I would never be athletic, that I would not have the opportunities to do the things other children did because of my disability. I could remember the doctors telling my mother that and how they wanted her to believe that, but I didn't believe that. I worked harder than everybody else at just being okay, and then I was able to turn that work ethic into being an outstanding athlete, which helped me develop the confidence, especially always feeling like I was living behind the eight-ball compared to everyone else.

Being told what I could not do also is how I got my first personal training certification. I was told, "You don't fit the standards of what personal trainers look like. You are not tall. You don't have blonde hair and blue eyes." Again, I didn't want their labels to define me, so I went out and got that certification anyway. I studied for seven and half weeks. We're talking about studying a 400-page textbook when I never even read a book of 100 pages. I then got my first opportunity to work at a place called New York Sports Club, a big box gym. When I got there, I was making $7 an hour, working four-hour shifts totaling $28 a day. It would take me up to 3 hours to get to work and cost me $20 in commute, leaving me with just eight bucks at the end of the day. Nonetheless, I worked my ass off, and I became one of the top trainers there within 90 days because I had to, not because I wanted to. If I didn't become a top trainer there, I would have been starving and would not have been able to take care of my grandmother.

I share all of that with you because without understanding the humble beginnings, you wouldn't know the ingredients that were necessary to help me stand on stages with some of the top thought leaders and be the confident man you see today.

One final thought. I always get asked, "Rahz, you make going through challenges look easy, how do you do it?" In all honesty, it was something I learned from my grandma. She taught me that what didn't break me made me stronger. You see, she was a beautiful woman from Montgomery, Alabama who had no education, never moving past second grade, but she told me that as long as I kept moving forward, I could be successful in life. She said if I kept moving forward, I would find someone who loved me and cherished me. She said that if I kept moving forward that it did not matter what the obstacles were ahead of me; I could overcome them as long as I got up every morning and prayed to God. This was downloaded into my brain because not only did she say it to me, but I saw her live it. Now let's learn about Greg, whose story will really resemble many fitness professionals' starting points.

Who is Greg Kalafatic?

For thirty years of my life, I've lived in Garden City, NY, where I had the honor of being the son of Marybeth Kalafatic and Alfredo Kalafatic. My mom was a nurse until she had her first child, and then became a stay-at-home mom to take care of four children while my dad took over his practice as a colorectal surgeon. For over forty years, my dad worked his ass off, waking up early and then coming home late at night. He really provided us with a very good lifestyle growing up. There were not many challenges that I can remember. As kids, we were given a lot. From private schooling to playing sports, to tutors, to participating in hobbies and other stuff we were interested in, he made it happen.

However, at 16 years old, I had to learn to become a man as my father went through some financial difficulties; the industry he was in started to change due to insurance companies.

It was then I first started to work, and I have not stopped since. I've always been involved with some type of work, whether it's in physical therapy, selling candy, catering, or even selling cigarettes illegally (don't judge me). While working, I did obtain a great education from attending private school (Chaminade) and then went to college (Hofstra), where I pursued my MBA in management. Unfortunately, I stopped four classes short because I had the mindset of there has to be so much more to life than me sitting in a class to get an education that I found useless. To this day, I have not gone back to school for my MBA, and I'm proud of the decision I made. You see, I've had that entrepreneurial itch since high school when I was selling candy. I did that for a year and a half before going on to sell cigarettes in college.

After this, I began looking for something online to do, which got me thinking about internet marketing. As you can see, I was a little all over the place, excited to keep trying new things. Following through on things was one of my biggest challenges. Starting them never was the issue, but finishing them wholeheartedly, not so much. I began to wonder what would serve as the kick in the ass I needed to break this habit, and that came at about 2005-2006 when my mom became terminally ill. I instantly became her caretaker. By this time, I was very privileged to have the ability to have a personal training job and going to school for kinesiology so that I could learn more about personal training. The personal training allowed me the flexibility to be home, drive to the city, and spend eight to ten hours with my mom during chemotherapy. I learned so much about my mom while spending this time with her. Personal training also provided me the opportunity to not have a job where I was sitting behind a desk, not to mention I loved lifting, and athletics was a big part of my life. Going back to school to improve my personal training also gave me the chance to learn more about the human body and what it took to teach someone how to transform themselves. Thus began the start of my journey as a fitness professional.

At the age of twenty-five, I decided to go ahead and do my first bodybuilding show. I thought of this as an opportunity to learn how to really transform myself so I could teach others how to do the same. This tip alone is gold. Too many times, there are people who are teaching others something they've never done before, but there will be more on this later. This desire to learn about the body combined with caring for my mom really started to put fuel in my fire to pursue a career in the personal training. My first place of work was at Equinox, where I first met Rahz.

The Meeting of the Brothers

Here we are at Equinox where I was already working for about a year when Greg joined the team. I was wearing the black shirt for full-time trainers while he wore the blue shirt for floor trainers. While I trained clients, Greg was responsible for mopping and putting plates and dumbbells away. I recall Greg having a little bit of a spark to him. He always tried new things and used pieces of equipment that most people did not use at the facility. I remember saying to myself, "This guy, he's really going after it." He seemed to just have a good spirit about him. For some reason, I've always been able to attract in my life good people in need of a little leadership. Being that I'm a Leo, I loved finding people and getting connected, but this did not mean an instant friendship with Greg. We were simply colleagues.

In The Voice of Greg

Rahz from my perspective when I first met him was different. Here was a guy who was walking across the gym floor with his earrings in, hopping over different things, shouting "Woohoo!" I instantly thought, *Dude, what's wrong with this guy's leg and why is he so happy?* When we started talking, a mutual respect for one another began to grow. Rahz was one of the top trainers there and always kept busy. He was that very strong, verbal, direct, and aggressive guy in a good way. While I had my father in my life—who was a great man—he was a very quiet man. He wasn't as strong a leader verbally as I saw in Rahz.

When I left Equinox, I was a struggling trainer who needed a bit of help; this is when Rahz took me under his wings and guided me along. I then remember when I went to Hawaii in March, Rahz had mentioned ideas of coming together. At the time, Rahz was leaving Equinox, making a declaration to one of his mentors, Jeffrey Combs, about creating his own business.

One day, it was raining, and Rahz didn't have a car. Naturally, I asked him if he wanted a ride home. I did not know this, but this left a nice impression in Rahz's mind about the kind of guy I was. We found an instant connection with one another and grew as friends; we both had to go ahead and become caregivers, Rahz caring for his grandmother for 15 years and me taking care of my mom.

I cannot forget the day when Rahz was talking about coming together. Wet behind the ears, I took it as if he wanted to be 50-50 partners, which I thought was fantastic, but initially, that was not the case. Rahz was the one with all the clients, and I was just someone who wanted to come on board and help while learning the sales and marketing side of personal training. I remember telling Rahz, "All I got is $2,000 to contribute, but I'm willing to work for free for a little bit." When I caught on to Rahz's vision, I knew this was something I wanted to be a part of and make a reality.

In The Voice of Greg (END)

Vision Behind Meta-Burn (The Start/Transition/ Breakthrough)

At this stage of the game, all we had was the belief in the saying "If you can believe it, you can achieve it." At this time, Greg and I were working together with the simple vision of creating the best personal training business that we possibly could so that we could impact one million people. While we had the vision, we did not know how we were going to make that happen, but it was great to have Greg on board. He understood the vision and was ready to work. We believed that if we got up early, stayed up late, and outworked everybody, we would win and never lose. With this mindset, we started to catch steam. People around us began to take notice as we integrated a lot of different things that we didn't even know we were doing. We were just ignorance on fire.

Next, we joined networking groups, going out there and speaking for free. I did lunch and learns, and whenever I wanted Greg by my side, he was there. When it comes to doing anything great with a partner, loyalty and trust is so important. Like he said earlier, he was not given outright a 50-50 partnership. At the time, what I needed more than anything was someone who was going to put sweat equity in the game. After that, we could talk about being partners.

When starting your business, trust is a hard thing to find. Especially for me, as the only person I trusted was my grandmother. However, Greg slowly but surely earned that trust, and we went on to do some great things within fitness. We were getting clients, and at one point we were independent contractors working out of a dance studio. It was while talking to Greg that he pointed out how much we were paying out, and we looked at each other saying, "We need to have our own place."

At this time, we transitioned from my grandmother's house to Greg's father's basement. This became our first headquarters. This would be considered the lean years in a trainer's business, but we actually had admins working for us. At one time, we had two or three people working downstairs with us in this crazy vision of doing in-home personal training, in-home nutrition, and a studio. We were doing it all, sometimes even having 14 one-hour sessions per day and repeating that day after day.

As we focused on doing, our vision board began to expand from one studio to two studios to three studios. Once again, we did not know how we were going to get there, but we understood that we didn't need to know the how—just the why. We applied what my grandmother taught me, to keep moving forward. Having Greg by my side saying that he would follow whichever way I went was huge. That's what a great right-hand man does. This allowed me to use my creativity. Before long, we had people asking how we were doing the things we were doing, which gave birth to our first official location in Locust Valley, New York in 2010.

This place was in a very competitive area, and we were doing pretty good before hitting some tough times in 2013. One thing we want to be real with is that everything was not an easy climb to the top. We did have some ups and downs along the way that included some tough decisions for our business. We changed business names, which hurt us short term, we moved 10-15 miles from our previous location, which cost us half of our clientele, and then we also made the decision to train only women, which cut our market in half.

All these decisions came with their consequences, but the setbacks also served as the set-ups to where we are today and what we have been able to build. In 2015, we opened our second location in Oyster Bay, and in 2016, we opened our third location in Mineola. Without these lessons, we would have just a bunch of fluff and theory to share with you in this book, not proven strategies that can withstand even the toughest times.

We also went on to put together Fitness Business Mastery mid-2016 as a result of all the things we did to see if these proven strategies would work for other trainers just like us. We felt it was one of the best ways to really hit our vision of impacting a million lives. If we could impact 1000 trainers who then impacted 1000 lives, we could easily achieve our goal. And this leads to why this book and why now.

What is the reason for this book right now?

If you've been in the health and fitness arena, you know far too well that a new book comes out every single day. From dieting to fitness training to how to build your business, it's as if it the red light at Krispy Kreme's is on when it comes to books coming out. If you add the fact that there are gurus who are entering the fitness industry space teaching how to make money and build your business although they've never been in the fitness industry nor had a successful business, you can see how the overload of information and skepticism can be at an all-time high. So with all these things into consideration, why would we still boldly enter the space of putting a book out?

In short, we want to see good trainers, good fitness business people, no longer get hurt or end up jumping on the bandwagon shift that is happening. Just because there are "gurus" out there taking up space, it does not mean there is no room for the people who are actually doing it. We wanted to share how to build a profitable business you love with struggling trainers and even trainers who were super successful but burnt out.

We have seen how this information has transformed us from a room in an apartment to multiple six-figure studios. We want to share the key strategies that got us there so you can optimize your business, too. We wanted to show you the 4 S's that you can utilize in your business in order to grow it and share how we utilized it to help our businesses grow. We are going to pull back the curtains and show the trials, the tribulations, and raw and relevant information that will help you uncover or pull out your greatest business. You won't hear stories about buying high-performance sports cars, pumping out alleged, fabricated numbers like how many seven-figure empires we've built, or a daily highlight reel of how "great" life is even when it's not. This is all going with the trend of what is happening in the industry today. We are presenting is how to create a lifestyle fitness business where you can experience the world, have a great time with your friends, and make a tremendous impact on the lives of others with your fitness business.

I know when you grabbed this book and heard the idea of a "One-Hour Trainer", that it would cause curiosity in your mind. We used this idea to capture your attention. From a marketing standpoint, it's important to know you can't impact anyone unless you have their attention. Whenever you're marketing, ask the following questions: How do I grab someone's attention? How do I get their curiosity up about what it is I'm offering?

When we came up with the concept of the One-Hour Trainer, these are the kinds of questions we took into consideration. This is more about building a team, leveraging systems, and being able to walk away from your business for a little bit so you can have a lifestyle while working in a business that you love. This is not about sitting on a beach with your laptop. You will have to watch your team, dial in your systems, and look over things, but it is not hard. You will put in the hours to make sales and market but you won't have to be the guy who has to burn the candle at both ends either.

If you no longer want to be that trainer that has to train clients from 5:30 am to 8 or 9 pm, we have a system in place to teach you how to build a team of loyal and trustworthy people to do that. We have systems in place on how to leverage your sales and marketing processes without being overwhelmed with how much manpower is needed to run these. No longer do you have to kill yourself to run your fitness business.

Who is the ideal person that should be holding this book in their hands?

This book is written for the trainer who wants to make an impact, make creative income for themselves, and put some certainty in their lives. They're beginners. They don't know much about systems, marketing, finance, sales, or customer service but they have a passion for changing people's lives with their message and their ability to help them create the best versions of themselves. It's for the intermediate who's been doing it for two to four years but is struggling and saying, "Shit, I'm a damn good trainer but I don't know how to attract more clients. I don't know how to attract my ideal client. I don't know how to stand out in a noisy market. What do I need to do to specialize so I don't generalize?"

Veterans, we did not forget about you. We do realize that there are people running businesses that look good on the outside but deep down they are struggling to make ends meet. Many veterans are one trainer or one mistake away from having to shut their doors. We want to help you not have to be fearful of having to cover a 5:30 am class or having to work until 11 pm every night again.

The goal of this book is NOT about pulling you away from your family and friends every night where they get fed up with you not being around and all you are left with are bills and a gym filled with equipment. We want to help turn you from a personal trainer to what we call a Pro.

Who is this book not for?

Since we talked about who this book is for, let's clearly identify who should run away from this book. If you are the internet marketing personal trainer who is looking to sit behind a keyboard and make money by putting up some ads and pushing a button, hoping to crush it, this book isn't ideal for you. While you could still learn from the sales and marketing aspects of this book, we discuss a different kind of business that requires leadership, action, and desire to help solve a problem for a market by leveraging the systems that we have in place.

I'll also add that this book is not for someone who does not believe in Kaizen. Kaizen is all about the mindset of constantly and always improving, not only as a skilled trainer but also as a person, a human being. We cannot say this enough; this book is about impact. You have to truly like helping people in order to absorb the contents of this book. If you're not one of those people—if you're looking for a microwave like success—this book is not for you. There is work involved. Your character will be developed from the stuff we share. This book is about helping trainers not just talk the talk but to walk the walk in front of and away from the cameras.

What can I expect to get as a result of listening to the story of you guys building this business model and sharing some of the strategies that has helped you to be able to live out this lifestyle fitness business?

You can expect to get some wind behind your sails in the form of inspiration and motivation from the real-life stories we share in this book. We are talking about raw and relevant stories that you can relate to no matter if you're a beginner or an expert. In addition, you will also get the step by step plan necessary to take the right actions on your visions and know how to keep it moving forward. You'll also get exactly how we troubleshoot some of our biggest obstacles so that you do not have to fall flat on your face when you face them. All of this will create the necessary momentum you need to go from vision to reality.

What Is The One-Hour Trainer and How Did It Come About?

The idea of the One-Hour Trainer came from an actual sit-down with one of our mentors, Ryan Lee, as we discussed some of the work we've done and the consulting we have done with some fitness professionals. As we talked about the different things that we do and threw things at the wall, Ryan asked Rahz, "How often do you train?" Rahz reply was, "Dude, for the last 14 months, I've been training one hour a week." It was like lightning struck as we all collectively thought, *That is what the concept of the book should be*. This is what the One-Hour Trainer concept is all about. It's about being able to create a business that works for your lifestyle instead of your business dictating your lifestyle.

Ideas such as if you're sick, your family is due for a vacation, or in our cases needing to take care of a loved one for weeks or months at a time, is where the concept of this book was birthed. The One-Hour Trainer is all about giving the fitness profession-al the ability and flexibility to run a business with a dedicated team that can support the scenarios previously mentioned. This does not mean you have to train only one hour. You can easily train five or ten hours a week, but it's all about leveraging your team, leveraging your systems, and giving yourself a little bit of your life back so you can do the things you love.

A lot of the time, trainers dream of running a fitness business only to be left with the nightmare of living broke, burnt out, and bitter—three B's that no one wants to be around. This kind of trainer finds it hard to make time for sales and marketing, and it's hard to truly care for their clients when they are all bent out of shape themselves.

This book is about putting all or your systems together to work together so you can have a business that is fruitful and profitable. We are talking to the trainers who do not have the desire to be a big box gym with 10,000-20,000 square feet and renting it out to others because they don't know what else to do with the space. *One-Hour Trainer* will show you how to make more money without having to take on more space. We will show you how within a 1,000 square foot studio you can generate a quarter of a million dollars to even $400,000 a year.

If that sounds like something you'd be interested in, let's take this journey together.

4 S's to Build a Lifestyle Fitness Business

We know who you are. Anyone who is a trainer started this career path typically because they wanted to help people. Perhaps you were in shape your whole life and wanted to share that with the world, or you were someone who was out of shape not fond of your life and wanted to share that feeling and experience of your transformation with the world. There are many ways you could have ended up here, but, at the core, a fitness business exists to help people get healthy and become the best version of themselves. In other words, it exists to make an IMPACT!

There is a glaring issue, however, that plagues many who decide to make this their business and life's work. The issue is the business is built around YOU. You are the person people want to train with, you are the face of the business, you are everything. The result of this kind of business, unfortunately, limits the number of people you can truly impact. And it also leaves you with absolutely no independence or freedom. If you're lucky, you can have a day or at the very least a few hours of that day to yourself.

So this begs the question:

How do we IMPACT more people, and make more INCOME without sacrificing INDEPENDENCE?

This is where the *One Hour Trainer* philosophy was born. It was born out of a need to help trainers increase their income, impact, and independence so they can enjoy the business they created and do it for as long as they want. Hence the term "Lifestyle Fitness Business."

The One Hour Trainer Lifestyle is built around what we call

the "4 S's". These 4 pillars will help you build the business you dreamed of and not a business you grow to dread.

Here are the 4 pillars:

1) How to SPECIALIZE so that you create a premium service

2) How to SELL so you can attract your ideal prospects and turn them into lifelong customers

3) How to SYSTEMIZE your process so you can deliver world-class service

4) How to SOAR so you can duplicate this process to expand or take your services online as another source of income.

Let's look a little closer at each one of these:

Specialize

This is where we develop your character and uncover your "Million Dollar Message" so that you can break free of the chains of being a commodity and turn into the premium service that the market has been looking for. When you build the character deep within you, the message that you are sending becomes more specific and focused. This allows you to create better results, and you will become a micro-celebrity within your community.

Sell

This is where we attract your ideal prospects and Unleash Your Authentic Authority. This allows you to convert them into long-term raving fans. This is where you will learn the most efficient ways to market and how to connect to potential customers and clients so that you are no longer selling on the basis of proving yourself but rather interviewing your prospects to become part of your tribe and join you on the journey you are leading.

Systemize

This is when you learn how to create checks and balances in your business and Unpack Your Lifestyle Fitness Systems so that everything works properly. When you learn this, you will finally be able to run a leveraged business that will run like a well-oiled machine, whether you are there or not. When the system is well-oiled like this, you can deal with situations as they come up, and you will understand the best ways to move forward and continue to offer world-class service.

Soar

This is the point where you empower your team so that you are able to duplicate the process and have an impact on more people in the market that you are serving. As a leader, you must be able to communicate to those involved in your business, be available, and offer consistent direction on a regular basis.

The scope of this book is focused on the first three pillars because it takes time to develop the foundation, which is necessary before even thinking of how to Soar. When you are ready to Soar, we invite you to a complimentary 30-minute strategy call to review where you currently are, understand where you want to go, and uncover the roadblocks standing before your dreams. At the end of this 30-minute call, you will have complete clarity and direction of the necessary steps for you to grow your business to whatever level you desire. You can book a time on the calendar at **www.resultaudit.com**

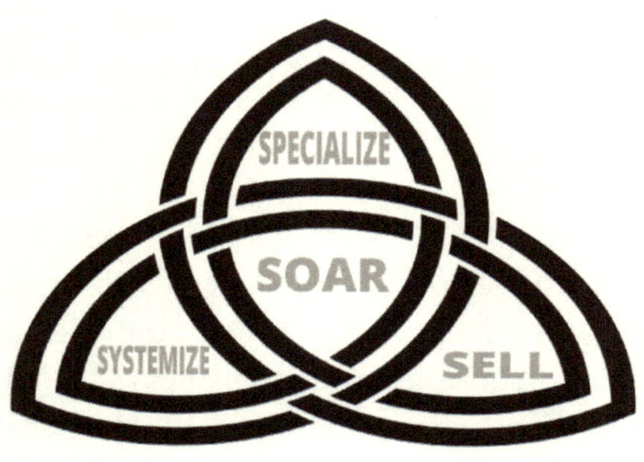

These days, the primary reason most fitness businesses fail is that they are servicing anyone and everyone. Somewhere along the way, trainers and coaches were told that you have the ability to help absolutely anyone that asks for it. While it's true that some people do have the skill set to help absolutely anyone they come in contact with, it doesn't mean you should try to save the world. This is the number one reason that these businesses fail; they turn themselves into a generalist, which means they have not positioned themselves as an expert in any particular area. They are doing the same thing that everyone else is doing. This makes them a commodity, which makes it difficult to demand the price they are worth. An example we like to share is the difference between a general physician and a heart surgeon. A general physician salary is on average $189,000, while a heart surgeon's median yearly income is $533,084. Which salary do you want? One of a generalist or one of a specialist?

To add insult to injury, most fitness businesses DO NOT know how to properly market—and more importantly: how to SELL. Marketing becomes YOU centric and why you are the best, while using manual tactics that not only take a lot of time but also don't have a clear way of measuring your ROI (return on investment). If any leads come through the doors from these outdated methods, you are anxious because leads are so inconsistent that you literally throw up all over your prospects with why you are the best. You then become submissive to their questions and lose control.

If you do happen to be lucky enough to convert a prospect into a client, it is all built upon you doing all of the work: from operating the business to customer service. You wear a variety of hats in the business. This leads to you becoming:

BURNT OUT

BROKE

BITTER

Your business ends up killing you, forcing you to leave this wonderful industry behind. However, that does not have to be your story. By the time you finish reading this book, you will learn how to incorporate the 4 S's into your business as well as the 9 strategies that lead to an amazing 6 to 7-figure business.

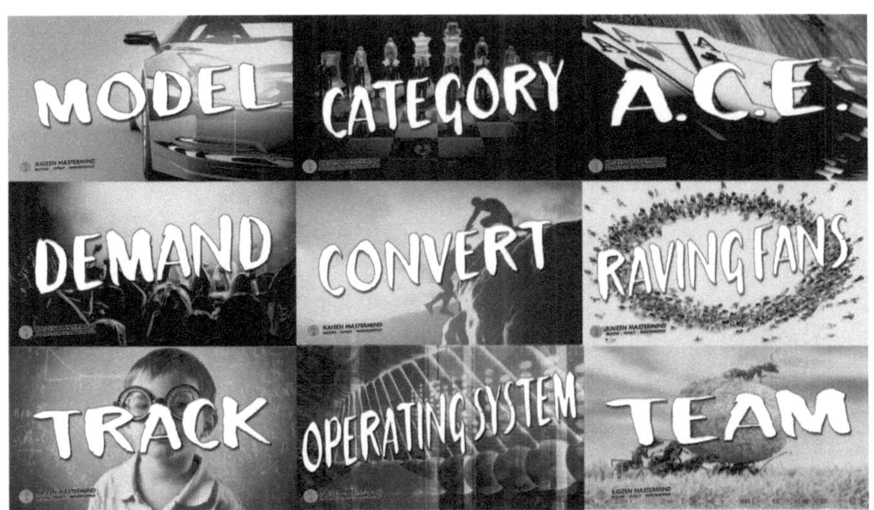

1. **Build Model:** Building your Model is all about picking the way you will service your market, whether it's One to One or One to Many. It is important to build this as the foundation before creating anything else.

2. **Own Category:** Owning a Category is crucial to specializing and demanding what you are worth. When you are able to solve the big problem of a market, they will follow you for a lifetime.

3. **Unleash A.C.E.** – Unleashing your A.C.E. is all about determining your messaging and how you present yourself to the market as an Authority, Celebrity, and Expert.

4. **Generate Demand** – Generating Demand is the number one challenge trainers have today in a world of clutter and distractions. This will teach you how to stand above the rest to get your message out there.

5. **Drive Conversions** – Driving Conversions is the only way to keep a business healthy and thriving. If sales aren't being produced, the business is dying. This will teach you how to get someone to raise their hand and ask to become a customer.

6. **Create Raving Fans** – Creating Raving Fans is the blood of a business because it's easier to keep a client happy than it is to find new clients and ignoring what you already have. The lifetime value of a client and the power of referrals are key to this strategy.

7. **Analyze Tracking** – Analyzing Tracking methods is going through the 5 categories of a business (Marketing, Sales, Operations, Customer Service, and Finance) and reviewing the KPI's to make sure the company is growing in all areas. Without knowing your KPI's, you could be in for a big surprise one day.

8. **Design Operating Systems** – Designing Operating Systems is building out all the steps, checklists, and systems that help the business operate as a smooth oiled machine. We take you from guessing and doing the work over and over to a more systemized approach on how to do things in order to save yourself time, energy, and money.

9. **Leverage Team** – Leveraging your Team is the next step in growth once you nailed down the previous eight strategies. Hire too fast without having the other strategies in place, and you can find yourself bleeding. But if you implement them right, you provide your team a great home to shine, and they will provide you with a lifestyle fitness business.

10. **The Flight Plan** – The flight plan puts this all together by helping you create a 90-day roadmap to a creating a lifestyle fitness business you love.

Before we get into the meat of the book and the nine strategies that will help you create a lifestyle fitness business, we want to share an impactful story from one of our students and how these strategies have changed his life and business.

Sumair Bhasin, TX

Train Life Fit

https://www.trainlifefit.com/

https://www.facebook.com/TrainLifeFit/

My name is Sumair Bhasin, and I'm the owner of a fitness studio called Train Life Fit in Austin, Texas. We've been in business for the past three years and specialize in helping people feel less pain, move better, and experience a better life overall through holistic strength and mobility training.

At the beginning of our business, unfortunately, I was really struggling. I was a one-man show and had no idea what I was doing. You could say

I lacked direction. Everything sounded like a good idea to do so that is exactly what I did. Unfortunately, running the business this way was literally running me to the ground. I was surviving on no sleep, waking up and training clients while struggling to take care of myself.

After realizing there was no way I could continue to operate my business like this, I decided to reach out to Rahz and Greg for some help. They were doing Fitness Business Mastery, and I thought I could learn a thing or two from them. Boy, did I.

They helped me install a foundation for my business. They knew I had large aspirations, but there was no way I could build it on a weak foundation, which is when they gave my business an audit. They looked at everything I was doing and taught me how to build the foundation that would help set up my business for future success.

Next, they helped me to dial down my systems so I could sell more and charge higher prices for my services. I was blown away when a simple conversation with Rahz helped me get twenty members at $210 dollars each. I was terrified with the idea of raising my prices, but with the strategies and techniques I learned through Fitness Business Mastery, I was able to confidently increase my sales and bring in more leads, all while getting my life back because of the systems Rahz and Greg helped me dial in.

The days of being stuck at $6,000 a month were now behind me. In the first thirty days of consulting with Rahz and Greg, I was able to pull in $10,000 for that month. With the continued support of Rahz and Greg, I've been able to consistently have $30,000 months and even hit a personal best of $35,000, all with just a studio of 900 square feet.

My business is now getting ready for the next stage: scaling the business. I'm excited about the idea of adding a second studio and adding more coaches so we can impact more people's lives for the better.

If you are looking to take your business to the next level, these are the guys to help you do it. I'm living proof that even a no direction, burnt out fitness business owner with the right coaching can get things back in line and build the ultimate lifestyle fitness business.

PART 1: SPECIALIZE

Chapter 1
Build Model

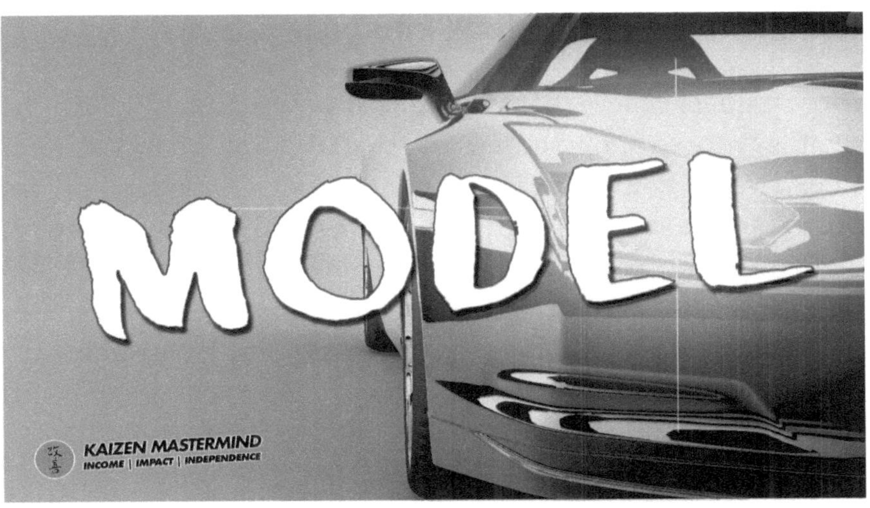

Have you ever spent a ton of money, time, and effort on something only to feel like it was a complete waste? We can think of how many times where a ton of effort, money, and time was put into having a successful event only for it to look nothing like I had planned. Unfortunately, this is a reality that many fitness business owners face. They go ahead and build a business that was designed to create greater income, greater impact, and greater independence like we talked about in the introduction but unfortunately did the exact opposite. The only thing you are left to say is "Why did I do that?"

When it comes to building a business, there are many factors that will be out of your control. Sometimes, that uncertainty can be the fun part of it. You can have an idea or might think of how it will go by following the advice of others, but nothing is for sure until it happens. While running a business, there are moments where it feels like you are walking through a foggy forest with many paths to choose from but not sure where they will end up.

What exactly is it about your business that scares you the most as you look into your future?

Most trainers believe that they can just wing it and walk through the foggy forest, hoping they will make it through to the other side. They're confused about how to navigate through the industry and exactly what type of business they should be building. If you don't have a clear vision, you become focused more on money and start paying attention and following the trends of what everyone else is doing. They start to have some self-doubt about what they want, so they end up selling their soul to the devil—and end up becoming like everyone else.

What you really want and need is total clarity so that you will be able to focus on your passion and have confidence that the business you are build is not only going to have an impact on thousands of people, but it will also serve you the type of lifestyle that you want. You want to start earning money doing exactly what you love.

That is why we have decided to open this book with the first strategy: *BUILD YOUR MODEL.* You must know your vision and be clear on where you want to go before you start building so that you can build your business on a strong foundation instead of the sand. Yogi Berra once said, "You've got to be very careful if you don't know where you are going because you might not get there." This section is all about ensuring you get rid of the fog and are clear on the path you're pursuing.

Before you do anything else, stop and think about what your business looks like and then ask yourself this question: *"What business model speaks to my passion?"*

Our fitness studios—Meta Burn Fitness—was built with complete clarity from the very beginning. However, early on, we fell into the trap of following trends. We changed our model a few times and restructured until we finally came back to what we initially visualized it to be.

Here are five principles that will help you build the right model that works with your passion and give you the lifestyle that you want:

1. Research business models

2. Design your lifestyle

3. Create a brand hero

4. Stand for and against

5. Sharpen your sword, not your pencil

Research Business Models

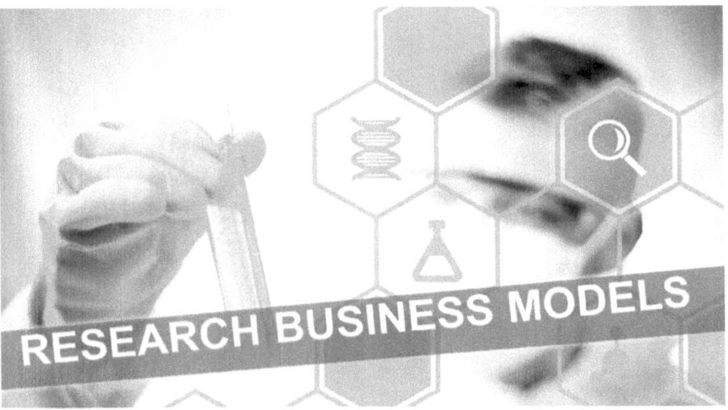

There are 3 business models you can choose from, and together, we are going to pick which one is best for you.

1. Private one-on-one

2. Semi-private

3. Bootcamp/class model

All three have their pros and cons. You can actually have all three in your business model, but you want ONE to be the sole focus of what your business offers.

Private One-On-One

This model is built around offering a premium service and having complete control of adapting your fitness and nutrition program to each individual. It's a powerful model that is easy to control, requires only a handful of leads to convert over into high ticket programs, doesn't require a huge space of overhead, and the results are typically better since you are able to serve each individual according to their needs.

The few challenges that arise with this type of model is you need to hire more coaches as prime time slots fill up, premium price needs to be high enough to pay out well and make a good profit, generally client upkeep is a bit more challenging as premium clients require a higher end service, and there's a need for more flexibility in scheduling as private clients expect to be able to schedule around their life instead of yours.

This type of model can position you as the authority a bit faster than the other models since you are offering a premium service. However, the higher your premium, the less of the market you are able to attract as it's seen as a luxury to have a private coach.

The private coaching model is awesome, but be prepared to serve on a high level.

Bootcamp/Classes

The bootcamp model is quite the opposite of private training. This model is built around a commodity service and becomes a bit more difficult to customize the program for each client.

The results typically aren't as good as private training as you don't get the chance to dive deep into understanding a client's life, and you require way more leads than you think to build a sustainable and profitable business. Typically, client retention is not as high, you attract more deal seekers, and you will need a larger space, which comes with a higher overhead.

From an operations standpoint, the more clients you have, the more problems can arise due to billing, customer complaints, or clients feeling like they are just another number.

On the flip side, if done right, this model can be very lucrative as you can generate more money per hour, it requires less staff, and it's an easy sell as this model doesn't have a very high price point. Marketing strategies like class passes, low barrier offers, or free trials can make this model easy to build and create a large client base as long as you have a good sales process in place. The energy is generally high as you have more clients working out together, and that social culture is easy to create since these clients are used to being in groups.

The bootcamp model can be a powerful model, but with the majority of fitness businesses offering bootcamps, it's seen more as a commodity and harder to differentiate yourself.

Semi-Private

The semi-private model is a hybrid approach to private training and bootcamp. The pros of this model is that you have good leverage in terms of dollars per hour you can generate, you don't need a ton of leads and clients to serve to have a lucrative business, there is a strong social culture created, and results can be on the higher side like private training. From an operations standpoint, you don't have to have a model that requires scheduling to be around each individual client. You set the schedule of times of operation.

The challenge with the semi-private model is that clients view it as having their own personal trainer in a small group setting, therefore requiring extra attention when they need it without a high price tag. Clients paying a mid-tier price point also want to have access to multiple training times in the day because if your slots are limited, they feel they are getting cheated. The other challenge is you need to be spot on with educating your staff or yourself to be able to handle a small group while providing that private training feel and being able to adjust on the fly. It takes a special individual to be able to control a small group while adapting the program to each person.

This model seems to have the strongest selling point due to its middle path of not requiring a lot of clients and being able to generate more money per hour, BUT it requires a special skill set to make it feel like private training and not getting caught up in being seen as the commoditized bootcamp model.

So, now you're probably asking:

"Which model do I choose?"

That comes down to which model you will fall in love with the most and can see yourself doing for years on end.

If it helps, we built Meta Burn Fitness based around private one-on-one training and made it feel like a small, family-oriented boutique. We just love that personal connection you can have with each client, and results happen quicker with that personal accountability. While our brand is all around a premium service, we do offer bootcamps as a special event a few times a year and have some semi-private options in the day for those who want the attention but just can't afford the premium one on one. We didn't build those two additional models into the business until we perfected the private model first.

Below is a graph we created to show you the differences between the models, amount of leads you would need, and number of consults in order to create $250,000 in annual business.

250K Training Business Plan				
Monthly Investment	Clients	Close Rate	Consultations (25% Lead Conversion)	Leads
$400	53	50%	106	424
		60%	88	352
		70%	76	304
		80%	66	264
$247	85	50%	170	680
		60%	142	568
		70%	122	488
		80%	107	428
$97	215	50%	430	1,720
		60%	359	1,436
		70%	308	1,232
		80%	269	1,076

There is no right or wrong answer, but once you choose the model that you know deep down you will love, the next step is to design your lifestyle.

Design Your Lifestyle

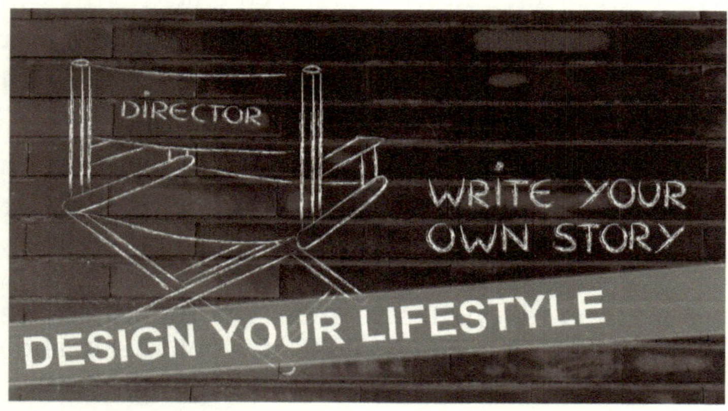

In order to reach a certain lifestyle of freedom, income, and impact, there are things you will need to start doing, continue doing, and stop doing. For this principle, we created a worksheet called the **Start, Stop, and Continue worksheet**.

When it comes to designing your lifestyle, you have to understand your strengths and weaknesses so you can serve your business at the highest level possible. This will also help keep you from becoming a burnt out, broke, and bitter trainer.

If you are just getting started, you must understand that you are going to wear multiple hats in the beginning until cash starts flowing and you learn how you can leverage yourself. On the other hand, if you are already established, you may still be wearing multiple hats, which is holding you back from growing.

The ***Start, Stop, and Continue*** worksheet is going to help expose what you are great at, what needs to be handed off, and what needs to start happening.

We wanted this book to be much more than just spelling out our philosophy and inspiring you. We wanted to give you nine solid strategies that you can use to create the lifestyle business you are looking for. Of course, you can just continue reading and skip all of the exercises. However, this book is going to have the most impact on you and your business if you take the time to work the short worksheets we have provided.

If you haven't already, go to **www.TheOneHourTrainer.com/worksheets** to download all the worksheets in one pdf to go along with the book.

Once you print out the worksheets, flip to the *Start, Stop, Continue* worksheet. Start with the first circle and take 2 to 3 minutes to list all of the things that you MUST STOP doing in order to have a lifestyle fitness business. This can be something small such as stop watching a lot of TV or stop designing your own flyers to the bigger things such as designing websites and funnels. Once you have taken the time to list the things you MUST STOP doing, you will have a list of things you can learn to outsource as you begin to have a more positive cash flow. This list helps you to see what your weaknesses are and gives you hope that one day you'll be able to delegate them all. These are also the things that you really don't enjoy doing.

Next, head over to the middle circle labeled CONTINUE. Take 2-3 minutes to list out all items and tasks that you MUST CON-TINUE doing. This may be because you're the only one that can do them or perhaps you have so much passion for these tasks that it is driving your business. List everything out right now because this list will tell you more about your strengths.

The last piece is the third circle labeled START. These are items and tasks that you know would change your business if you started doing them. This can be anything from getting more sleep, posting more content, meditating, or facing your fear of doing more public speaking. Take 2-3 minutes and write everything you MUST start doing to drive your business to the next level.

The beauty of this worksheet is you can fill it out every ninety days and find that each circle will change as you build a team or learn new skill sets that better serve your business.

Create a Brand Hero

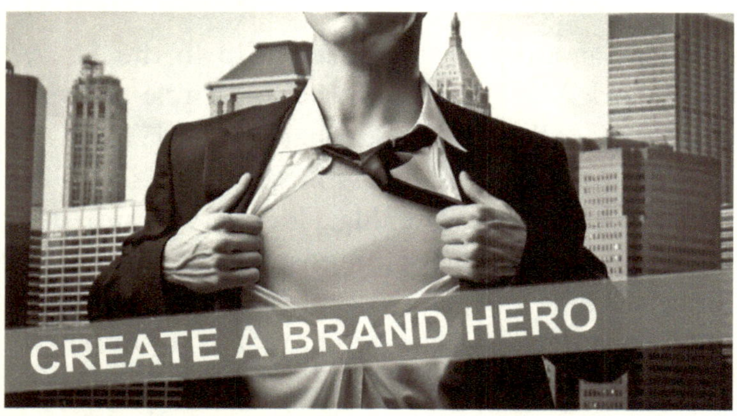

Now that you have selected the business model you want to build and you've designed your lifestyle, it's time to create your attractive character. An attractive character represents your business and is one that the market can become attached to as their leader. Don't overthink this.

Here are the various types of heroes to choose from:

1. <u>Leader:</u> Individuals whose goal is to lead people from point A to point B. In most cases, leaders share a backstory that is similar to their audience, so they know the challenges that their audience will face on their journey. Typically, the leader has already achieved the desired results, and the audience has come to receive help on that same path. You most likely have leaders in your life that you follow—whether you realize it or not—and this may be where you are most comfortable communicating with your audience.

2. <u>Adventurer:</u> Individuals who are curious but don't necessarily have all of the answers usually assume the identity of an adventurer and begins a journey to find the truth. Then, the adventurer brings back treasures from the journey and shares them with the audience. The adventurer identity is a lot like the leader, but instead of leading the audience on their journey, he or she gives them the answer.

3. <u>Reporter:</u> Individuals who have not yet blazed a trail to share with their audience but desire to typically assume the identity of a reporter. These are the ones who are going out to discover the truth. Individuals who assume this identity have talked with lots of different people and share what they learn with their audience.

4. <u>The Reluctant Hero:</u> Individuals who don't like to be in the spotlight and don't want any attention brought to their discoveries takes the identity of the reluctant hero. However, he does know that it's important to get out the information/secrets that he has, so he gets over his shyness and shares them.

For example, we have Coach Rahz "The Motivator" who is a natural born leader always leading from the front and by example. He is direct and straight to the point. On the other hand, Coach Greg, "Mr. Nutrition" is the reluctant hero who doesn't like the spotlight, but he has learned many things along the way and knows he has to find a way to share them.

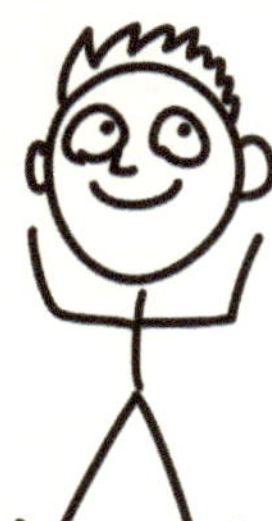

Stand For & Against

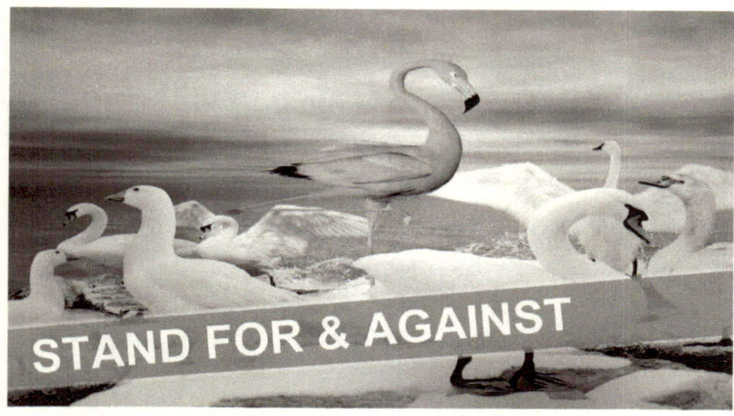

Now that you know what type of hero you are going to be and you have given yourself a name, it's time to clearly state what you and your business stand for and what you and your business stand against.

Remember in the beginning when we spoke about the first S,

which is specialize? Well, the number one way to clearly specialize and stand out is to let the market know EXACTLY what you stand for and against.

You want to draw in the people that you want to work with. You want them to be attracted to your message and follow you. On the other hand, you want your message to repel those that do not align with your business so that you can set a clear understanding of who you are, who you serve, and what you expect. Sure, this is going to piss a few people off, but for every person that you piss off, you'll attract 10 others who love your message. Also, this goes perfectly with the quote that says, "If you do not stand for something, you stand for nothing at all." By not choosing something, your business ends up representing nothing.

The easiest way to do this is to pull out your worksheets and flip to the *Stand For & Against* worksheet. Take 5 minutes for each section. On the left, list everything you stand for and then on the right list everything you stand against. Don't over think, just start writing.

When you finish and reread both lists, what you stand for should put a smile on your face, and what you stand against should give you such disgust that you are happy to tell your market what you don't stand for.

Sharpen Your Sword, Not Your Pencil

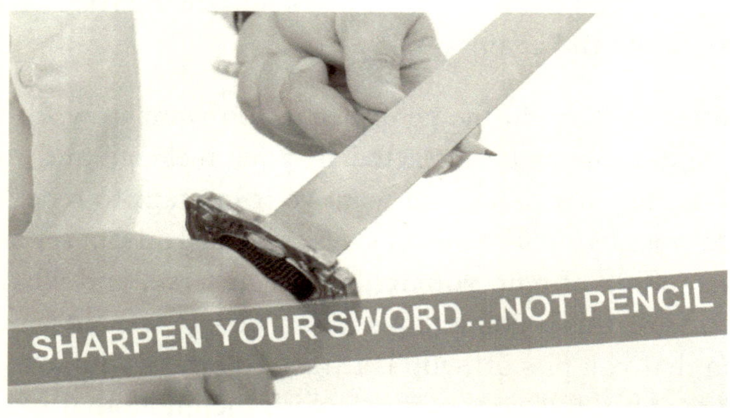

This is a metaphor for mastering things that are productive skills (sword) not time wasters (pencil). Your sword is the things that make sure you are victorious and successful, and your pencil is the things you do because they are easy but don't have a big impact on your business. The great personal development guru, Jim Rohn, might have said it best, "Don't major in minor things."

All too often, most trainers focus on becoming the best trainer possible to the point that that they forget about the fact that there is a whole business component to actually serving people that need your skills. When starting out, getting certified, reading fitness and nutrition articles, and attending workshops are your sword, but when all you do is avoid marketing and selling because you feel that you have to be the absolute best in your market, those actions start to become a pencil.

Knowledge without action is a waste of time.

Learning and applying things that will actually take your business to the next level are the swords you need to sharpen. They are things that have a learning curve, take patience to learn, and create an impact on your business. Here are a few items below that can be seen as your sword that you need to sharpen:

1. Initial training certification
2. Initial nutrition certification
3. Social media marketing
4. Building funnels
5. Public speaking
6. Joint ventures
7. Creating lead magnets
8. Create content with calls to action
9. Collecting testimonials
10. Hiring and delegating

Here are a few items that can be seen as your pencil that you need to put away:

1. Taking 10 different certifications at once
2. Putting flyers up
3. Making random posts on social media
4. Talking about yourself with clients
5. Mistaking productivity for bullshitting on social media
6. Creating a brochure website
7. Hiring cheap help
8. Sleeping in
9. Pitching your service without rapport or connection
10. Handing out business cards

Become a master swordsmith, not a pencil sharpener.

Congratulations! You just completed the most important strategy for creating a lifestyle fitness business. Without this foundation, you are building your business on sand, which eventually will erode and crumble. With the foundation in place, you are ready to now **OWN YOUR CATEGORY.**

Chapter 2
Own Your Category

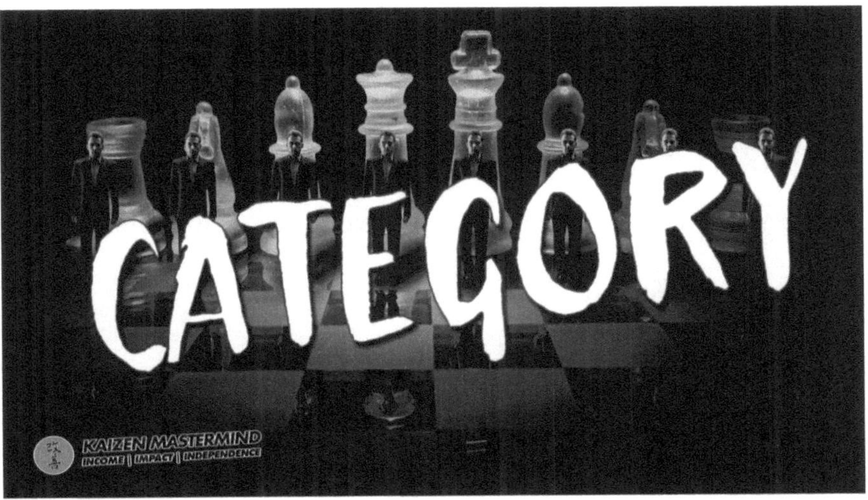

I have a question for you. It's Christmas time and you need to go buy some toys for a little niece or little nephew; where would you go to buy them? Chances are your choice would be Amazon, right? What if I asked where you rented your movies from when you want to kick back? Chances are, you might say Netflix. The reason why the majority of us would think the same things is because these companies understand what it is like to "OWN A CATEGORY." It's the same kind of power we would like to go ahead and help you cultivate. There is tremendous power when you have T.O.M.A. (Top of Mind Awareness) with your potential clients.

When it comes to owning a market, most trainers are afraid to focus on one submarket because they alienate everyone outside of it. When you learn how to be good at everything and serve everyone, you will find yourself in the commodity market where people undervalue your services and will always negotiate with you. When you create a category of one or master one market, you will be seen as the expert and can demand premium rates no matter the model you choose.

So we have a question for you:

Who is your ideal market?

When you answer that, you then have to ask yourself:

1. Can they afford it?

2. Do you like working with them?

3. Have you gotten them results before?

The main frustrations trainers have is that they are attracting the wrong people because they have not clearly stated who they are. They take in clients that are literally zombies that have no excitement or interest to change. When you start attracting everyone, you have to learn to control the chaos and soon have amateur status stamped on your forehead. The ultimate fear is that you start dreading going to work.

What you really want are ideal clients you could see yourself having a beer with. Know how to serve them at a high level, and you become a local celebrity to them. This is what we call "Living the Dream."

Let's dive into the five principles that will help you **OWN YOUR CATEGORY**.

Know Your Avatar

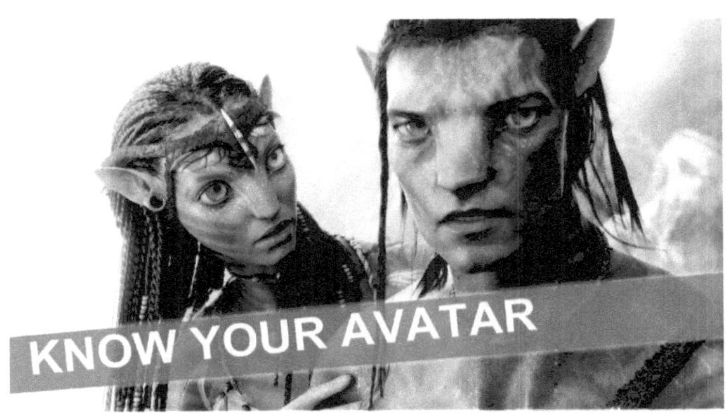

If you have been reading about marketing and sales, chances are that you've heard a lot about this lately. The challenge is that most of the time, trainers don't really get very deep into who their avatar is. They choose the one market that everyone seems to target: the 35 to 50-year-old woman that wants to lose weight. The problem is, this is way too general, and you end up competing in the weight loss industry with every other fitness related business.

To solve this problem, we have created a ***Customer Avatar*** worksheet that you can download from **www.theonehourtrainer.com/worksheets**

Even if you think you know exactly who you serve, fill this worksheet out so you can fine-tune things.

Start in the middle by filling out all the basic demographic information like age range, marital status, occupation, etc. Once you finish that, start in the top left box and work clockwise. Get as specific as you can with your avatar's goals, values, challenges, pain points, sources of information, and objections and role in the purchase process. Take ten minutes to fill out the worksheet to the best of your ability. Do that right now then continue with the book.

Done? Are you sure you didn't just skip that step? Skipping this is no different than your clients skipping a warm-up.

If you did skip that worksheet, it's only preventing you from creating that lifestyle fitness business. We created these worksheets to help grow your business—not keep you busy.

As you clearly define who your avatar is and understand where they are and where they want to go, your message to market will be so precise that your ideal client thinks you are speaking directly to them.

Don't just blindly put out content or copy and paste. Truly understand your market, connect, and show them you understand what they are going through. This can be seen as hard work, but they are spending their hard-earned money with you, so it is a fair exchange.

True Reality

Now that you detailed out your avatar, it's time to dig a little deeper. Yes, there is another worksheet, but it will literally take you five minutes. Before we get to that, let's discuss what we mean by true reality.

If you've seen the movie *The Matrix*, the main character, Neo, soon realized that his reality and what he saw in front of him was just a façade. It was a mask hiding the truth. The truth was his reality lived inside the Matrix, which controlled everything.

Your ideal clients are no different. One reality for them is their desire to lose weight or to be fit, but that isn't always their true reality. The 'lose weight' or the 'be fit' goal is the out loud conversation they are having, but there is also a conversation they aren't having out loud that you want to know about. It's that other conversation that when it is not addressed that leaves ideal clients feeling defeated and unsatisfied. If you understood that private conversation your ideal clients were having, do you think you could help them more?

Damn right you can!

Let's use an example. Let's say you described your avatar as Mary who is forty-five years old with three kids and is a stay at home mom. Since she had kids, she put on forty pounds and hasn't been able to shake it off in the last two years. She reads *Women's Health* and realizes her problem is she is fat and out of shape because she doesn't have the time to do anything and is very self-conscious about her body. Every day, she body shames herself and is unhappy with what she sees.

Do you think if you market to Mary with a 12 Week Transformation that she will buy right away?

Yes, it's possible. However, what if she sees an ad or flyer of yours with a woman in her 20's who is fit and looks sexy in fitness clothing? Along with that, it states that for your 12 Week Challenge, she must come to the gym 4x a week and follow your diet plan. It can sound like an obvious solution. Unfortunately, over the last two years of Mary's life, those forty pounds have made her self-worth tank, and her kids consume all of her time, so she doesn't think there's any way at all that she can lose the weight and dedicate the time to your program.

Chances are, you'll lose Mary's interest—as well as that of others like her—when you market like that because your posts, emails, and flyers are geared toward women who are already confident or love working out but just want to lose a little bit of weight. This is why it's critical to fully understand the reality of your ideal prospects.

Once you know a prospect's urgent, expensive problem, it's easy to sell them a long-term fitness program. First, understand their reality, then quantify the cost of the reality, and last, list out the emotional impact of that reality if they stay there. Go to the worksheet labeled ***Avatars $10,000 Problem*** and fill out the three categories listed. This will change how you communicate to your market, and you will see how they will respond more positively to your message.

Get this worksheet done in five minutes, and we will see you at the next principle, **FINAL DESTINTATION.**

Final Destination

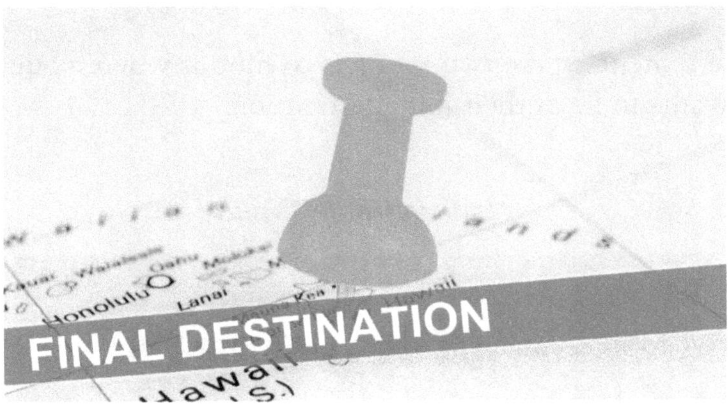

You know who you will serve and what their reality is, but that's still not enough. You have to understand where they want to go. What's their ultimate destination? It's a like a joy ride except there is no joy because you don't have a clear destination established.

For instance, this book is geared toward the personal trainer who is a great technician, but they don't clearly understand the marketing, sales, finance, operations, and customer service components of a business. They know what they have can change many lives, but they fear scaling their business will make them burnt out, broke, and bitter.

Ultimately, their final destination is how to create a lifestyle fitness business that allows them to impact way more lives, create more income for their family, and have more independence to enjoy life while running a business. This book is geared exactly toward that trainer, not the big box gyms or the studio owners that have multiple studios and are crushing it (unless you find yourself doing everything in your business).

Dive in deep to where your clients want to go. Take out the worksheet called ***The Prospect Journey,*** and from your previous reality exercise, write in their reality of where they want to go from where they are currently.

In one sentence, take two minutes to fill out where your prospect wants to be at their final destination.

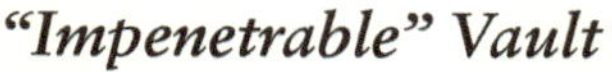

"Impenetrable" Vault

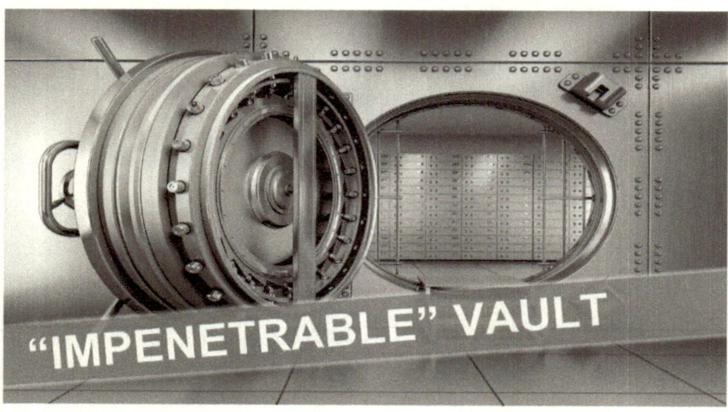

Now that you figured out the reality of your prospect and you know where they want to go, what's missing? This next principle addresses a blind spot that is rarely addressed, instantly builds a connection with your ideal clients, and gets them making a mad dash to work with you.

This principle is called the "IMPENETRABLE" Vault because even if a prospect has an outcome they want to achieve and you speak to that, they still may feel that they can't accomplish the end goal. They don't yet have the trust in you or themselves to get over the roadblocks in their way. When you can present content to your market that addresses where they are, where they want to go, and how to overcome the roadblocks in between, you earn the trust of your ideal prospect.

You can't just say "Hey, I'm pretty cool. Buy my shit because it will help you." How will you help them solve that underlying voice they have inside that is telling them this stuff won't work like all the other stuff you've tried before?

On the same worksheet, ***The Prospect Journey***, fill out the middle section called 'Roadblocks.' List as many things your prospect feels is a roadblock standing in their way from achieving the ultimate destination. It doesn't have to be perfect or 100% correct. For two minutes, brain dump everything you feel the roadblocks are before you move on to the next principle.

Milestone Therapy

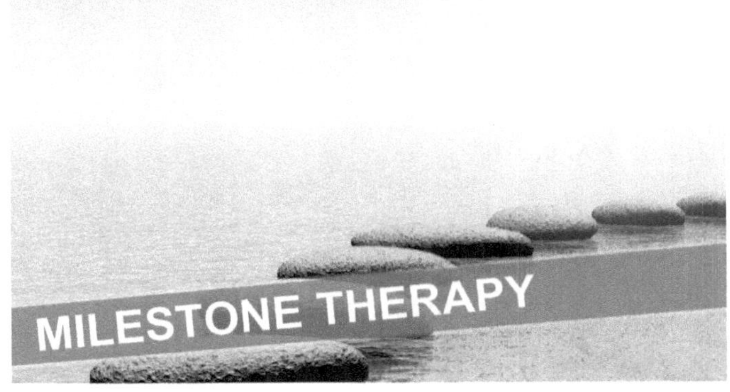

By now, you are starting to develop your attractive character and voice to your ideal market. Over time, it will evolve, so be patient and keep putting your message out there even if you feel no one is listening short term.

This principle "Milestone Therapy" is crucial in gluing this all together. You want to put this principle into play ASAP. Understanding how to celebrate milestones in a client's journey with you is crucial. Once you get to Part 2, Sell, and Part 3, Systemize, you will learn more steps on how to attract and sell clients and how to serve them with an onboarding process, but you want to start brainstorming ways you can celebrate your client's success before you start picking up more clients.

For example, at Meta Burn Fitness, here are just a few of the things we have in place:

T-shirts that say, "Lost 20 lbs."

a success wall of before and afters

a hall of fame wall

video testimonials documenting clients' journeys

welcome package when they make the decision to join

texts when they accomplish something new

thank you cards

gifts for when they refer clients that sign up

$5 Starbucks gift cards for their birthday

What are some things you can implement into your fitness business right now that if your client received along their journey would make them feel a part of your community and never want to leave? You can just think out loud or write in a blank space of this book a list of things you could do or give your clients that don't break the bank but gives them that "therapy" that you actually care?

Congratulations! You just finished Chapter 2 and didn't make this book another dust collector on your shelf. By now, you should have a much clearer understanding of who you want to serve and how to own your category in the market.

Our biggest question to you is:

Do you become the queen or do you stay the pawn?

In chess, the pawn—although an important part of the game— often gets sacrificed for the greater good and is seen as a low-value piece, while the queen dominates the board, moves effortlessly, and has a high value on the board. Commit to being the best in the market you want to serve!

With the category you want to serve in place, you are ready to now **UNLEASH YOUR A.C.E.**

Chapter 3
Unleash A.C.E.

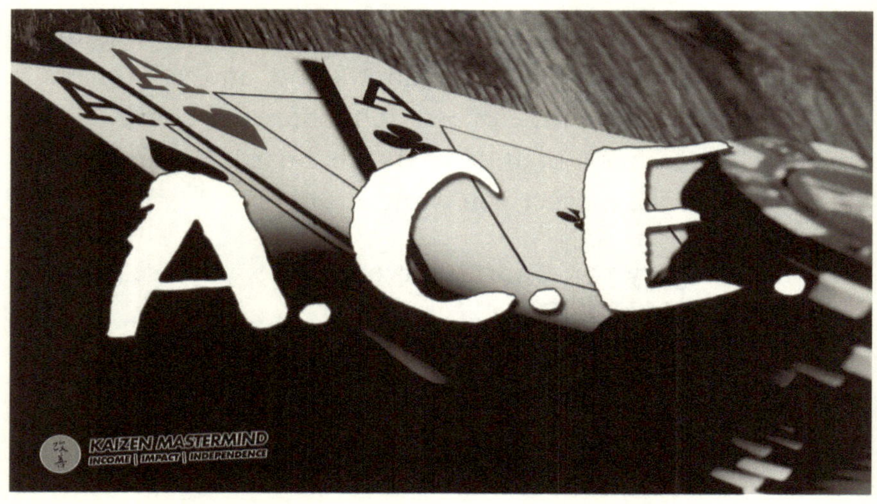

If you ever held a deck of cards in your hands, and someone asked you to go through the deck and pick out which card holds the highest value, most likely you would pick the ace. It's the one card that stands out above all others. It doesn't contain a number or a picture. It stands alone.

This is one of our favorite chapters because it's what makes the business a lot of fun and allows you to demand the prices you are worth in the market. This strategy allows you to dominate so you never have to worry about closing your doors while watching your competition dwindle.

A.C.E. stands for Authority, Celebrity, and Expert.

The worst thing that can happen to you is to be seen as your title "Personal Trainer." Let me explain before you start debating why we are wrong. When the word personal trainer became known in the 90's to the general public, it was seen as this luxury or person that a celebrity or professional athlete would hire. But today, the word personal trainer has become commoditized. Don't believe us?

Look at the top paid fitness celebrities or mentors that you look up to. They are seen as icons, not personal trainers. They made a shift by understanding how to solve problems, put out more content than anyone else, and show their leadership in the market.

So, our question to you is: *Who do you want to be seen as in your market?*

The problem is you aren't getting paid what you are worth, you are obscure to the market, and you are like a zebra that just blends in with the bunch. It's like auditioning for a movie or singing competition. You walk in confidently and feel you are way different than everyone else only to have your dreams ripped away from you by the judge telling you that you are just like the others and don't stand out. That's exactly what the fitness market does every day to trainers.

What you really want is to be paid a premium for your services, show up in the spotlight, and create a category of one to those you serve. This is your ticket to Hollywood!

Let's jump into the five principles that will clearly set you apart from every other trainer, so you can dominate the market.

Authority Website

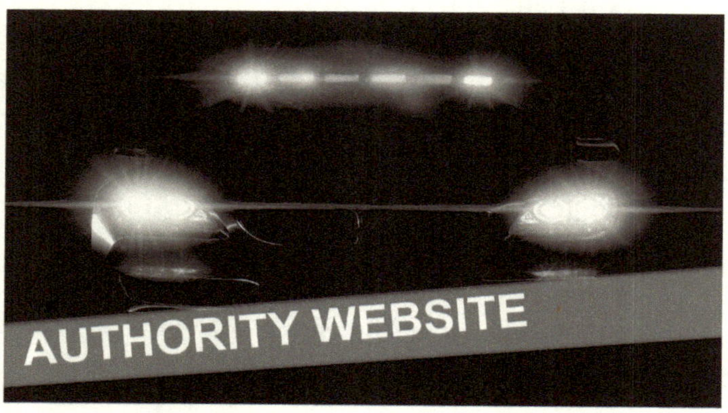

We have to admit, websites aren't the most fun to build because they can take a while depending on your developer and how well they get your vision. A little secret, but we advise you don't follow this path. Our website got hacked into twice over a 9-month period of time, so we just didn't rebuild one a third time. We went about 18 months without having a website because we were dominating Facebook with our ads and converting at a high enough level to have record breaking months. We finally have our website up and running, but if we would have just invested a little extra time to rebuild that site earlier, we probably would have had sales from our site as we did in the past. We don't have everything perfect yet, but at least you get to learn from our experiences ☺.

There are four pages that you must have on a website so that it converts high and doesn't act like one of those boring brochure sites.

1. **Free Gift** – This is something that is low commitment/risk on the prospects side, yet it solves a problem they are having and provides a simple and time-saving solution, like a checklist or hack they can implement right away. What's popular for our

market is our 7 Day Slim Down Meal Plan or Body Type Diet Guide that they can opt into right on our website.

2. **Training/Webinar** – This is more of a time commitment and requires a set meeting time. The higher the commitment, the lower the conversions you might experience with a cold market, but as you build your list, you can always send them back to this part of your website. A webinar is an in-depth training that solves more problems but dives deeper and allows for more interaction with your ideal prospect. Once you find a webinar that converts well, you can make this section of your website into an automated webinar.

3. **Four Part Video course** – This is a bit less of a time commitment than a webinar and allows a prospect to watch videos on their own time, but still requires them to learn more information. This section of the website is great for teaching three different topics, and the fourth video sells them on why they need your help and takes them on a journey in this video course.

4. **Case Study** – This page on your website is all about relating a story that touches your ideal prospect. It allows them to visualize what their life could be like through one of their peers. This draws out the emotion and builds you up as the local celebrity.

These four pages combined will generate leads as you sleep and automates some of your marketing as you continue to put content out to the market. There are several ways you can build a website. You can hire a developer to create an HTML site which you own and have good SEO, but you have to maintain and protect it, or you can use a platform like we do for our sites, which is in the resource area at:

www.TheOneHourTrainer.com/worksheets

Your USP

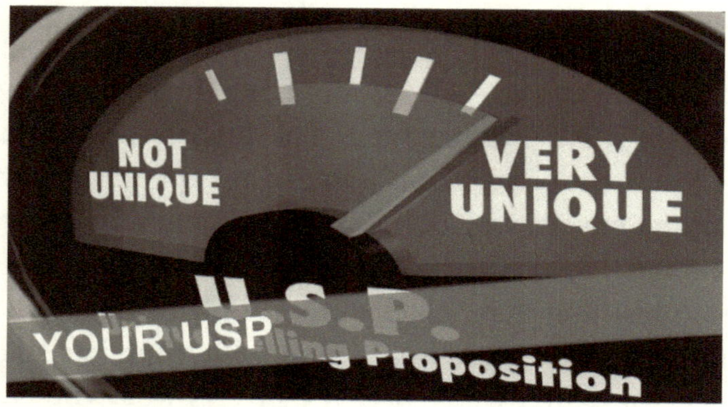

You may have seen these letters thrown around often in business. USP stands for Unique Selling Proposition. This means what's so unique about you that will compel someone to give you their hard-earned money. To take it one step further, even if you are unique, how do you get someone to trust and believe in you?

There are three types of beliefs to gain trust.

First, a prospect must believe in you as the leader to be able to help them get where they want to go. Many times, it can be difficult to convince someone in a 30 to 45-minute consultation for a first-time meeting. That's why it's crucial you have so much content out in the market that people are warmed up to who you are, what you stand for, and the fact that you care.

Second, a prospect must believe in themselves to get the desired result. This may seem like it's out of your control, but it's not. As you release content, whether written, video, or audio, address the most common objections your market has or talk about how one of your clients used to have this belief that nothing would work for them because they tried everything... until they tried your program. It's the perfect feel, felt, found overcoming objections formula. The more of this type of content you put out, the more your prospect will have higher hopes they can actually change.

Third, they must believe in your product delivering the results. If you are not putting out written or video testimonials or having your clients leave reviews, you are missing the boat big time. The only way to prove that your product works is for their peers to talk about how your product/service changed their life. Your words alone won't work; they expect you to say good things about your own services.

As you can see, most business books teach you just to state your USP. That is like being the Seattle Seahawks on the one-yard line in the Super Bowl. If you want to put the ball in the end zone, you have to put actions behind the three belief patterns so your USP can score.

Author a Book

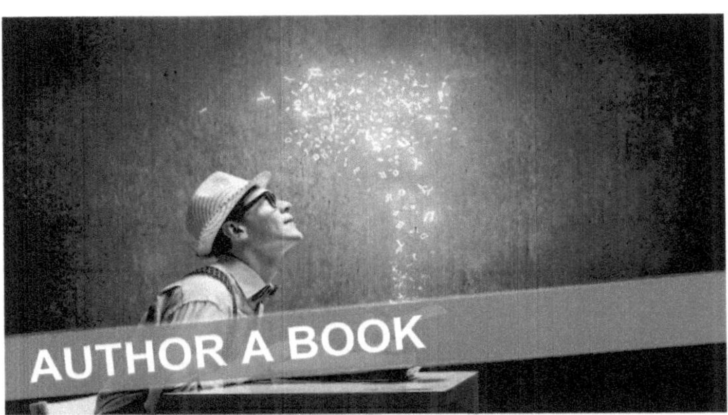

Writing your own book is one of the fastest ways to bump your authority and expertise in the market you serve. It's not as complicated as it sounds, and we will show you the easiest way to get it done.

Just think of the power of your own book. When you have a problem that you want to solve, what do you generally do? You'll post on social media about it or you'll google some solutions about it. 9/10 times someone will mention a book that can help or a google search will show you the title of a book that matches your problem. Next, you buy that book. Most times you take it as truth and start following that person who wrote it.

Instantly, that person is credible to you even if you never met the person.

We want to show you how you can literally have your own book scripted out in seven days. It will take a bit longer to edit, create a design for the cover, and set up ways to self-publish it, but within the 7 days, you will have all your expertise out on paper. You ready?

Step 1: Map out the main problem your book will solve

Step 2: Break down your solution to this problem in 5-10 chapters

Step 3: Either ask a trusted friend who is great at interviewing or hire a third party to interview you. Have them ask you questions regarding each piece of the solution plus add some of your background to provide context.

Step 4: Get the audio of your interview transcribed at Rev.com

Step 5: Hire an editor to take these transcriptions and put it in an order that reads well and sounds professional

That's exactly how we put this book together plus *The Menopause Success Triangle*. We hired a third party to first interview us on the biggest problem this market is facing, what our solution is, and brainstorming some ideas. On our second call, he grilled us on each topic until we had about two hours of content. Then, his editor organized it and we approved and made changes where necessary. If you are looking for someone that can help you with this process, we can connect you with our guy if this is something you want to move ahead with.

Borrow Authority

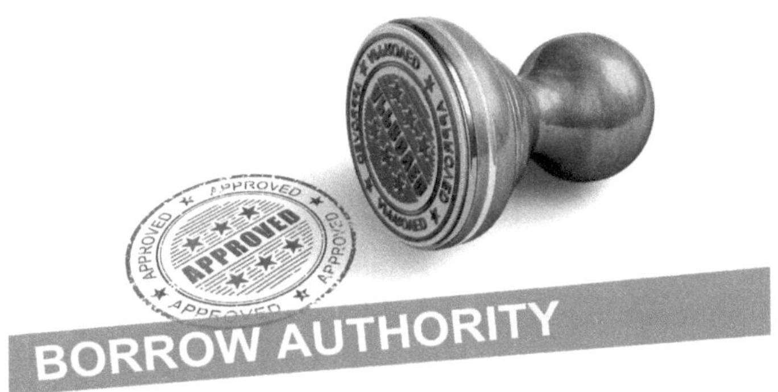

I know it sounds cheesy, but it works! You literally can borrow someone else's authority as you are build your own. Ever see that guy or gal who is literally everywhere and takes pictures with celebrities or experts in your field? Or better yet they just interview everyone that is an authority to the market they want to serve, which automatically links them to that status.

It's a necessary step in order to raise your perception as an authority figure in the market, and it's the easiest thing to do. Now we are not telling you to go take a picture with someone higher than you, tell people you are longtime friends, and make up a story to borrow authority. That happens way too often, and it's not within our values to teach that.

The best approach is to see how you can add value to the authority figure you are trying to borrow from plus add value to your market.

Here are the five best ways to borrow authority ethically and effectively from someone that will help level up your perception of the market.

1. Speak for Free – Speaking for free or even paying an authority figure to speak on their stage gives you a strong presence in front of their market and yours. The power of speaking is priceless as you have no idea how it will impact your business down the road, but there is always someone watching you from the crowd that will connect with you on a deeper level. The perception is if this authority figure invited you on his stage to speak to his audience, there must be a major value that authority figure sees in you, and now you are seen on a similar playing field.

2. Write for Free – Writing a blog for a successful blogger in your industry, articles for organizations like Huffington Post, or even posts for influencers on social media can get you recognized as an authority very fast. The key is you have to be a great writer and understand how to deliver value via the written word. If you are not great at writing, take courses on storytelling and copywriting.

3. Start a Podcast Interview Series – This is super easy to set up, and most times when you reach out to other authority figures, they are very open and happy to do an interview with you for your audience. You don't need crazy mics or software. You can literally grab a smartphone mic, record on your phone, and use an app like Anchor to get your podcast out. Make sure to pick authority figures that complement what you do and will add value to your market.

4. Host Your Own Event – It can be scary to host your own event. Trust us, we've done many events for our studios and for our consulting practice, but they are not as hard as you think. As long as you do a great job in building up the suspense via different marketing avenues and have a great hook for your audience, they will show up. Inviting an authority figure down to your own event links you two together, and your audience will see you in a different light.

5. Start A Master Class Series – A master class series is an in-depth training that teaches your market how to solve a problem over a series of trainings. You can invite one authority figure or multiple authority figures that are experts in a certain area to a master class series either for free to your clients or for a small front end offer out to prospects in your market.

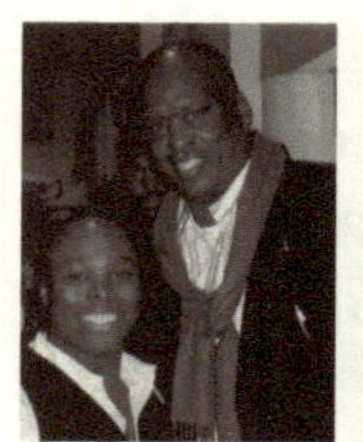
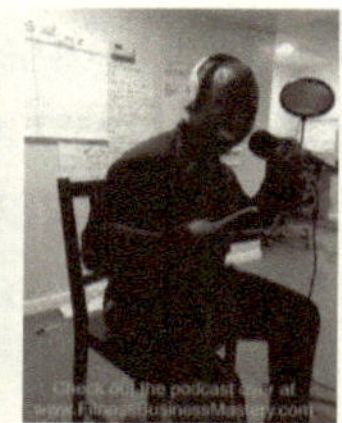

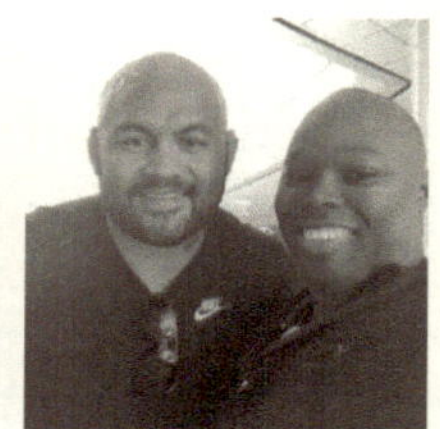
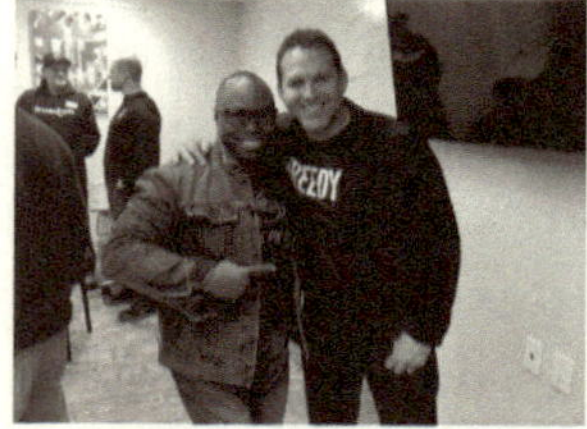
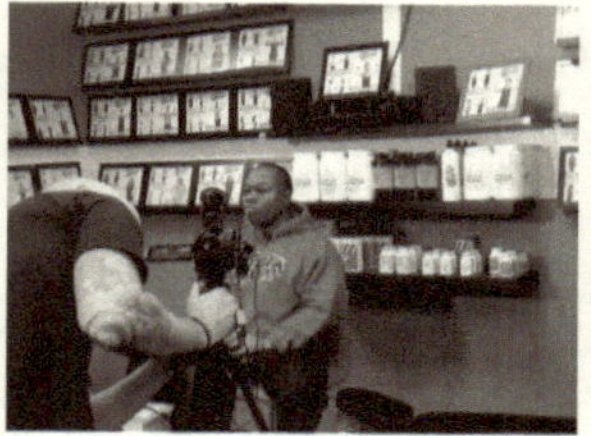
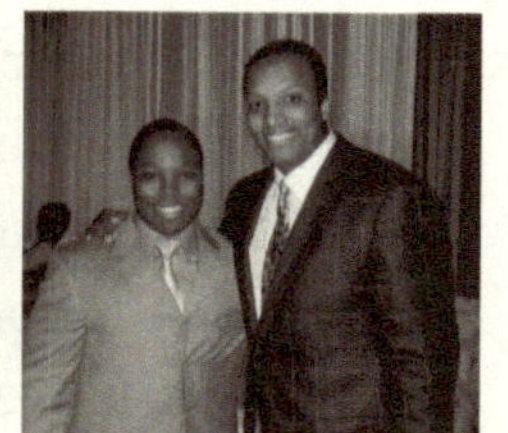
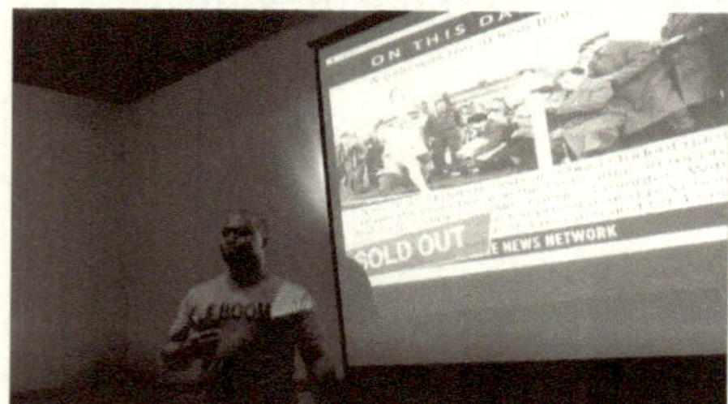
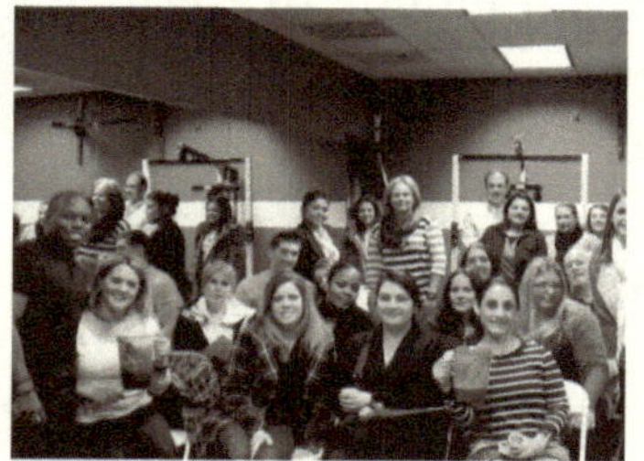
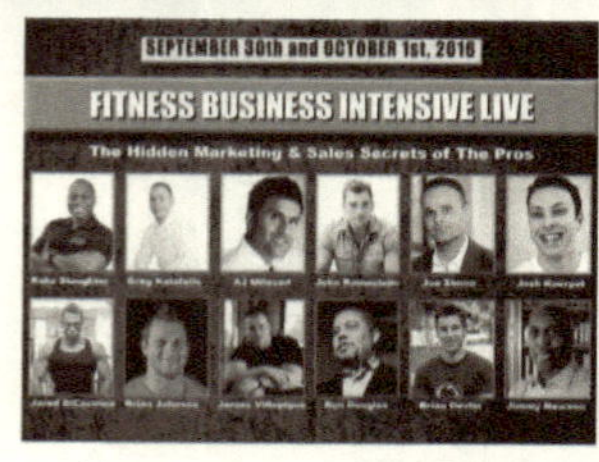
SEPTEMBER 30th and OCTOBER 1st, 2016
FITNESS BUSINESS INTENSIVE LIVE
The Hidden Marketing & Sales Secrets of The Pros
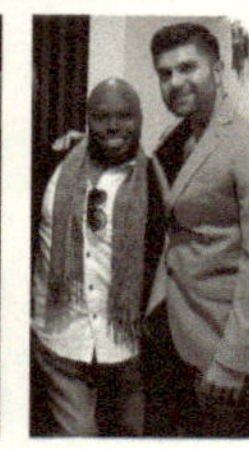
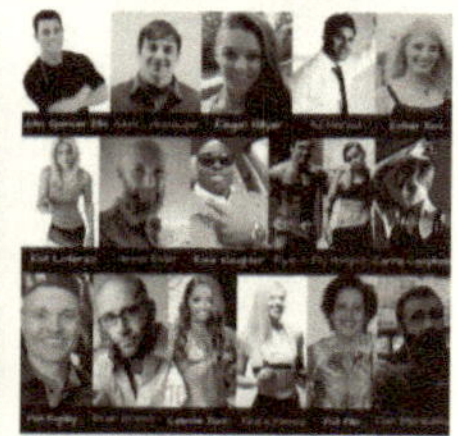
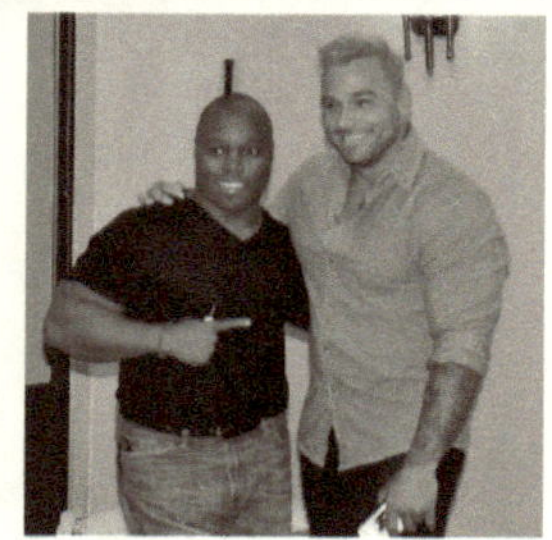

Have A Mission

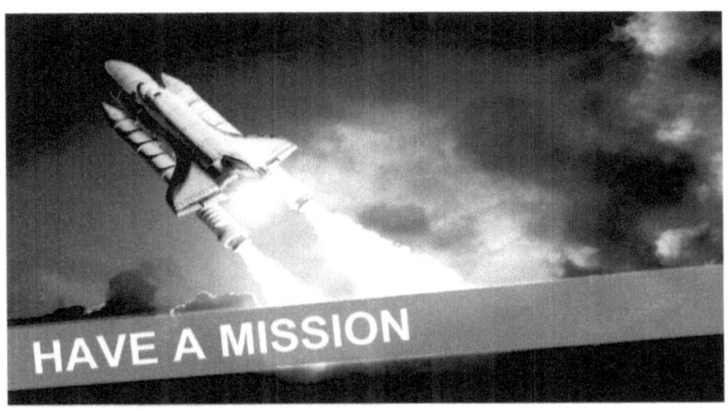

What is the cause that you are championing? Every person that you admire who is a dominant figure in a market typically has a mission that they have created or adopted as their own. Having a mission goes in line with what we talked about earlier about what you stand for and what you stand against. That would be a great worksheet to revisit to help put together what your mission is. If you can put a combination of what you stand for and what you stand against in one cohesive thought, that would be a great recipe for what your mission should be. The mission is a great way for your ideal clients to know what you are about. Who do you stand for, and how do you plan to serve your market? Those are important elements for any market leader.

For example, our mission is to create 1,000 One Hour Trainers with our products and mastermind services in order to impact 1,000,000 people with their health and fitness. We knew we couldn't impact that many people with our studios alone, so we had to equip Fit Pros with the knowledge, strategies, and systems to impact their market in a big way.

Take five minutes to write down what your mission is. DO NOT be corporate and generic like you have been taught in school. It can be a sentence or a few sentences. It doesn't have to be perfect.

Congratulations, you just finished Chapter 3 and are one step closer to becoming an authority in your market.

Our biggest question to you is:

Who do you need to become in order to be seen as the authority in your market?

Understanding the key elements to Building Your Model, Owning Your Category, And Unleashing Your A.C.E., you are now ready to go into Part 2 of the book which is **SELL** and you will start off with **Generate Demand** which is all about marketing.

PART 2: SELL

Chapter 4v
GENERATE DEMAND

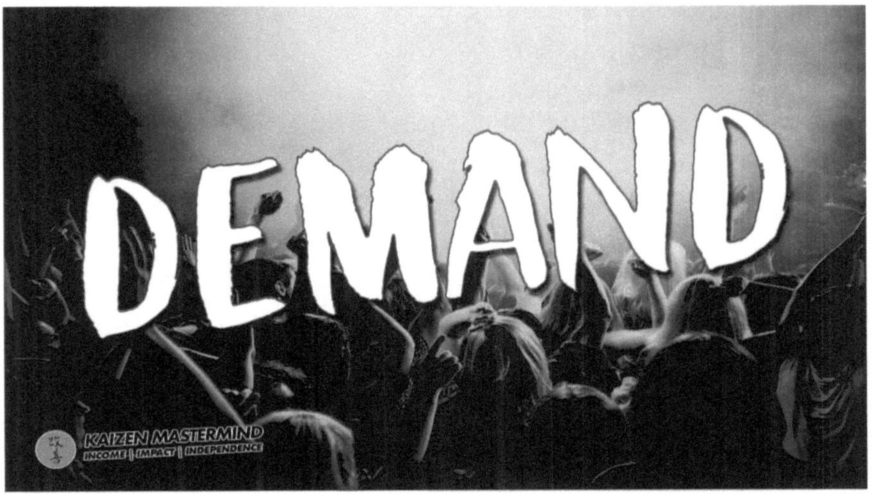

When's the last time you went to a baseball game?

We are Mets fans, but we found ourselves at a Yankees game because a buddy of ours invited us to the Legends Suite. It was an opportunity we couldn't pass up. Now being completely infatuated with business, all we did was hang out for 40 minutes before the game and started to observe various ways the ballpark made money and how things were structured.

We watched the lines wrap around the stadium, parents' pockets emptying on buying swag, food, and beer, and the sheer excitement of each fan wanting to get in to see the game start.

It's a frenzy of fans waiting for that opening pitch.

That's what we want for you: to be able to drive that DEMAND for your services and create raving fans that love what you do.

But can I tell you a secret?

Most trainers and studio owners live by a hope, a wish, and a prayer. They are reactive instead of proactive, and they sit back hoping someone will call them or walk in the studio. A wish, a hope, and a prayer is not an effective strategy. What if we could change all of that for you?

Imagine getting 50 qualified leads to your business in the next 30 days without having to make cold calls, attend networking events, hand out flyers, or run a lunch and learn workshop.

How would being able to push a button and have leads pouring into your business change it?

I bet it would change your life. And no, we are not some cheesy marketers that will have you believe you push a button and leads just give you money. There is a whole process that needs to happen before you push that button and a whole process you'll learn in the next chapter on how to sell those leads into high ticket programs.

But, it's a simple process if you just take a few minutes to follow along.

The problem is most trainers and studio owners are dry as f@ck and have no leads coming in; they are burning cash on old-school marketing tactics and losing clients without a plan of how to replace them. That's an exact formula for closing your doors and losing your business.

If you take this chapter seriously and not just a section you breeze through, we will show you how to get a boatload of leads so you can feed your piggy bank and attract new clients to have a thriving business.

Are you ready for the five principles to turn this all around for you?

The Prospect Journey

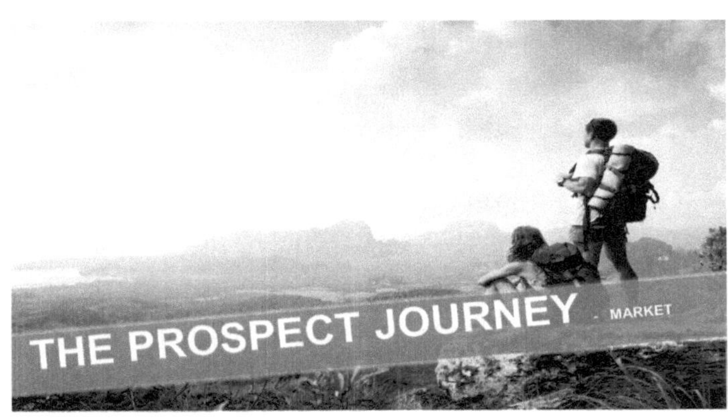

There's a reason why we lead the book with building a model, owning a category, and creating A.C.E. Doing the worksheets in those sections is crucial because it will clearly define your message to the market, so if you have not done them, do them now.

I know you are an educated and smart coach that wants to make a difference because you wouldn't have picked up this book otherwise. That's why it's crucial you understand your prospect's journey because a woman going through menopause is going to have different life experiences, challenges, and changes in her body than a 30-year-old working woman that is career-focused not family-oriented.

Imagine if you could really get in the head of your market and know what keeps them up at night and the conversations they are having in their head.

Dive deep into your ***Prospect Journey*** worksheet if you haven't already.

If you want to go the extra mile, you can take it a step further by going out and interviewing complete strangers in the market you want to serve—or even people you know—and ask them a series of questions of what they like, what challenges they face with their health and fitness, what their dreams and goals are, what they read and watch, what part of their body they'd change if they could, and the one thing always on their mind about their body, health, or fitness.

Now the key is to make this feel very safe and comfortable but also to reward them with something to give it their all. Maybe 1-2 personal training sessions as a thank you. Not only will you get some instant leads, but they just told you how to sell them if they come into your facility or you go to their home. If you are going to guide a whole market to victory, you have to know their end goal and have things in place to overcome the challenges along the way.

Speak their Language

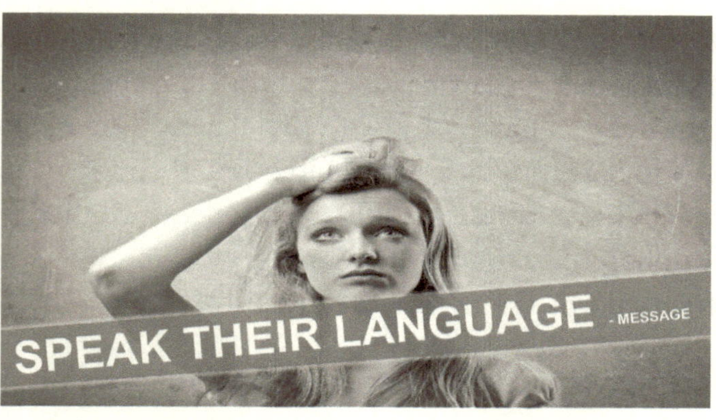

Ever read the book, *The Game* by Neil Strauss? It's straight up all about pickup artists and how there's this underground market of men and women that want to learn how to pick up the opposite sex. Go pick it up, ONLY after you finish this book. Doesn't matter if you are a happily married man or a woman who thinks that's disgusting to teach people how to pick up others using NLP or psychological tactics.

Read it for the storytelling genius behind it and to see how that underground market has their own language when speaking to each other. If you spoke their language, you were just like them, and you could sell them anything you wanted.

The days of just blanketing the market with generic health and fitness tips are over. It doesn't work and has zero appeal.

Who the f@ck wants to read another article on why carbs aren't bad for you or why you should drink more water. Is it factual? Yes. Does it grab the attention of your market? Most likely not. You want to speak the language your market is speaking so they feel you are just like them or at the very least you understand them.

For example, Rahz is known as the menopause expert in the local market. How does a black male who body builds, walks with a limp, and is dyslexic become known for something he's never experienced in life?

Well, he authored a book on the topic, interviewed top doctors, held a menopause summit, and put out content acknowledging the issue at hand and the solutions behind it. So, he can put out an article the same as you do on why drinking water is important, but if you make it generic for everyone, and he shows how hydrating helps with these menopausal symptoms, he will win every time when it comes to driving new leads.

Don't follow the trends of buying email software that gives you content to send out to your list or simply copy and paste the generic articles going around social media. Pretend you are speaking to your ideal client when you are writing, recording an audio, or shooting a video. It will help you craft a message that targets them directly.

Dominate One Platform

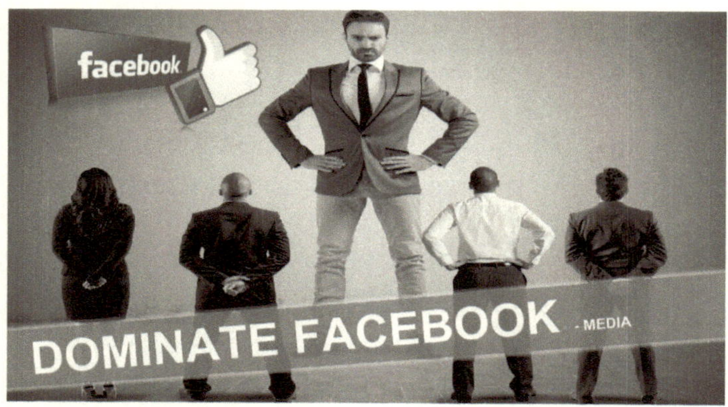

What happens when you tell a brand-new client that they need to diet, exercise 3-5 days a week, stretch, meditate, prepare all their food, do extra cardio, maybe try yoga, get a massage, journal how they are feeling, and stop drinking?

They are either going to stay silent and fail miserably in your program, or they are going to ask for a refund shortly.

Why?

You overwhelmed them with way too many things and made it feel impossible to achieve their outcome.

It would be the same outcome if this section told you to create accounts for YouTube, Facebook, Snapchat, Twitter, Instagram, Active Campaign, and on top of all that, join a networking group, create mailers, hand out flyers, and do workshops in order to be a successful trainer.

You would flip us the bird and move on to the next book that taught you one simple thing to do.

We are huge fans of Gary Vaynerchuk. If you don't know who he is, go watch his Daily Vee or listen to his podcast. He's all about being everywhere and anywhere and mastering every platform. He's a rare businessman that is hard to replicate.

So, we want to keep this simple for you and dominate one platform. We suggest Facebook to start. In fact, we will show you an easy strategy with Facebook if you are brand new to advertising on it. In the worksheet handout you download-ed at **www.theonehourtrainer.com/worksheets,** you will see a checklist called the ***Client Surge Checklist***. That will walk you through a simple and easy to use Facebook strategy to start getting new leads. As you learn the platform, we have more advanced strategies we teach at our 1 and 2-day sales and mar-keting workshops, but for now, let's keep it simple. Read the next two sections before you start using the checklist.

One Entrance

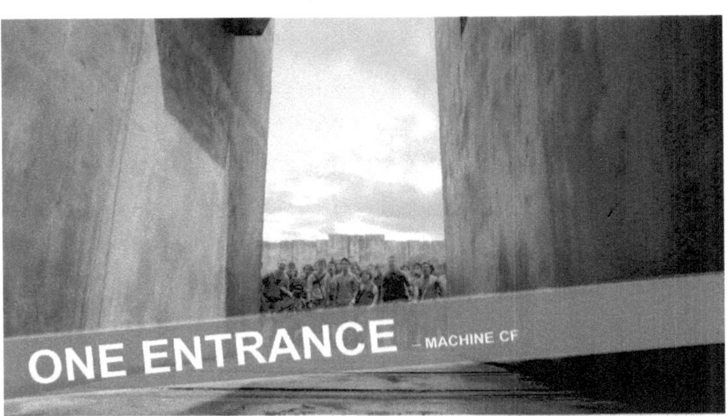

Ever been to the restaurant chain The Cheesecake Factory? The moment you sit, they slap down this encyclopedia of a menu with about 1,000 choices of drinks and food. Unless you have been there before, it's a very overwhelming feeling and hard to make a choice.

This is the exact feeling you want to avoid when a prospect learns about your business. The principle of One Entrance drivees your prospect down one path to focus on. You have your authority website that gives them everything if they find you online, but when it comes to driving traffic or using paid advertising, you don't want to send them to your website where they have multiple options to choose from.

For our business, we use a funnel building software that helps us create that one path that clients go through. If you want to learn more about this software, head over to **www.FunnelsForFitPros.com**.

The software allows you to easily create funnels (micro websites) by just dragging and dropping different elements so you have a headline, a video or image, some benefit copy of what the prospects get, and a simple opt-in box where they give you their name, email, and their cell number (this is optional).

Let's use an example. Our market has expressed the uncontrollable food cravings they have, so we created a small guide called Combat Cravings. Instead of saying go to my main website and download the guide somewhere on the page, we created a sales funnel solely dedicated to the Combat Cravings guide and how this one thing will solve the challenge of food cravings.

In copy on the ad pages in the funnel and the thank you page, all we talk about is solving that one problem, their food craving. You get them to take one action and allow them to feel confident and develop trust that you have the solution. They don't need to know about your blog, your about page, or how to contact you just yet. Once they are in your funnel, you can email them different pieces you want them to see along the way.

Can you see the benefit of why you want to make this a simple path for your prospect and why it's not a smart idea to send cold traffic to your main website?

You can register for a 14-day trial of the funnel software we use by going over to **www.FunnelsForFitPros.com**

Micro-Commitments

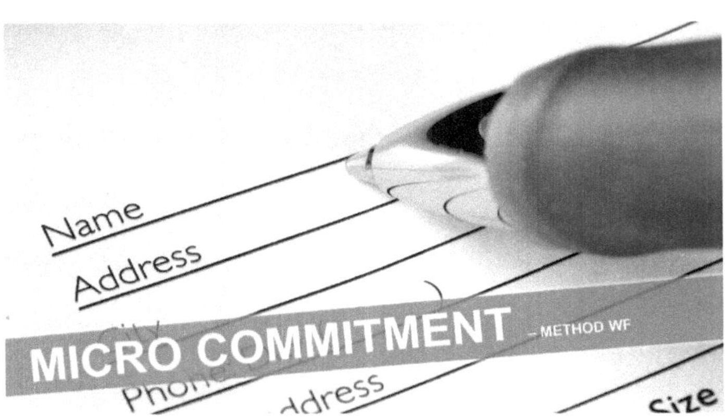

In a sales consultation, if you can get a prospect to answer YES to several of your questions when you ask for the close, what are the chances they will say YES to that last question?

It's pretty damn high when you do sales right and get them to commit to saying YES to your questions that you will convert them. That will be discussed in detail in the next chapter, but for now, I want you to take away what's happening when they say YES.

It's called Micro-Commitments.

A prospect is committing to small pieces along the way giving you buying signs that they are interested in what you have to offer.

This comes back to your funnel from the previous principle on One Entrance. When they come to that one page with your one solution on it, if they fill in their name, email, and more importantly their number, that's a micro-commitment that they want what you have. In other words, they are saying yes.

Imagine if on the next part of that funnel there was an application page where you thanked them for downloading your guide to solve their problem but you have a special program that will take them to the next level, which could be your 6, 12 or 24-week program. Do you think they might fill it out? The odds are yes!

Here are two amazing things that happen when you put that application on the thank you page (a cool resource to make the application is called wufoo.com):

1. An application is a more in-depth form, asking open-ended questions which signify to the prospect that you are a serious program and want to learn more about them.

2. It presents an image in their mind that you don't accept everyone, and they have to prove they are a good fit for the program.

If they fill that out, how serious do you think that prospect is about getting started with your program?

They are very serious, and chances are when you call, they are excited to hear from you. It's another micro-commitment you got from them that is low risk and required no additional time on your part.

There are more advanced strategies for adding more micro-commitments we teach in our workshops, but for now, this is all you need to get started.

The personal trainer or studio owners that get the most micro-commitments from the market will dominate the local area in a short period of time.

CASE STUDY

Holly Drayton, TN

Better Body Fitness

http://www.betterbody.fitness/

https://www.facebook.com/BetterBodyFitness/

Holly is a veteran in this industry with 22 years of experience. She has had her studio in Smyrna, Tennessee for the last three years. Being in an industry for so long, one is bound for ups and downs throughout the process.

Prior to this, Holly owned a very successful Fitness Together studio in a very high-end area with a partner. It wasn't uncommon to have a prospect walk in and drop a few thousand dollars for personal training. She built up a strong presence in the area and was rocking it with the results for her community.

Towards her 8th year with the Fitness Together studio, the energy started to shift with her partner and a current client. Long story short, greed kicked in, and they planned to force Holly out through a loophole in the contract. The client had money she wanted to infuse into the company, and part of it was buying Holly out of her partnership.

With her hands tied and the contract not in her favor, the only thing she could do was accept the offer.

Imagine that. Investing all this time, energy, and money only to get screwed in the end from a disloyal and greedy partner. Emotionally, that can drop someone to their knees and make them question, "Do I still want to do this?"

But I don't think you know who Holly is. She's a do-whatever-it-takes type of gal. Even though this situation hurt her and set her back, she was able to dust herself off and open a hybrid 3,000 sq. ft studio in Smyrna with both bootcamp and personal training services.

The biggest hurdle with this move was the area's median income. It was $52,000 per household. This was quite a flip in financial terms compared to her previous studio in a very wealthy area. So, her strategies had to change in order to build up her new company Better Body Fitness.

One of the main challenges when we first started consulting with Holly was getting leads through the door and handling the objection of "It's too much money."

She expressed her frustrations with a previous marketing agency who got her leads, but they were unqualified leads that lived 15-30 miles away from her studio and were inconsistent. The agency made this promise of getting her leads, but they forgot to mention how they were ripping her off by not targeting her ideal audience.

The first thing we did was set up a custom 6 Week Challenge Sales Funnel with Holly and a Facebook ad campaign to target her ideal audience.

Let's just say Holly no longer has a challenge getting leads, and her sales conversions and prices increase as she creates that authority in her market. She is kicking ass and changing women's lives in her local area.

Just in her first day launching her new 6 Week Challenge, she got 22 leads that were within 2-4 miles of her studio and heavily qualified due to the nature of the sales funnel. She spent on average of 0.89 per lead and the total cost for the day was $19.77. This blew her mind because she'd never seen this type of lead flow in her career for this type of marketing spend.

It would be great if we could maintain that type of lead cost and lead volume throughout her entire campaign, but it's nearly impossible as her reach is pretty small within her local area.

To sum this up and tie it in with this chapter, over the last 84 days of her campaign, Holly generated 279 leads at an average cost of $5.54 per lead and total campaign spend of $1,546.94 and has put in over 50 new clients into her bootcamp program, many of them signing on for 6- and 12-month contracts after.

By creating that local authority and targeting her ideal clients through the Facebook ad platform, Holly is now able to reach lead flow that most studio owners and trainers dream about but are unsure how to do.

With the One Hour Trainer book, now you have the same blueprint Holly has to become super successful even in low-income and low-populated areas.

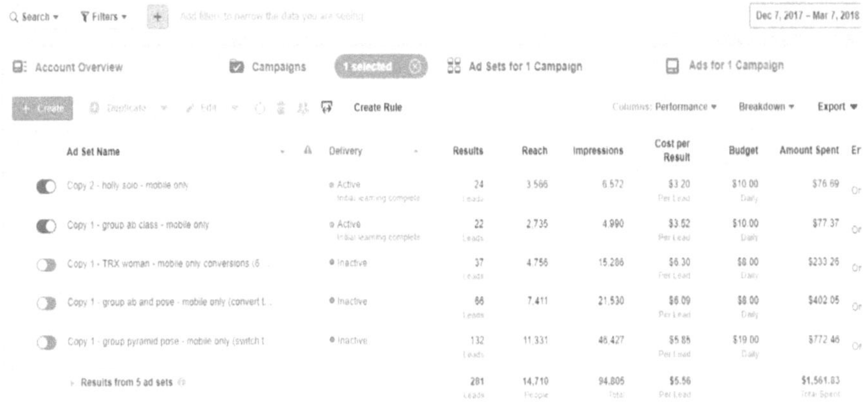

Ad Set Name	Delivery	Results	Reach	Impressions	Cost per Result	Budget	Amount Spent	Er
Copy 2 - holly solo - mobile only	Active / Initial learning complete	24 Leads	3,566	6,572	$3.20 Per Lead	$10.00 Daily	$76.69	Or
Copy 1 - group ab class - mobile only	Active / Initial learning complete	22 Leads	2,735	4,990	$3.52 Per Lead	$10.00 Daily	$77.37	Or
Copy 1 - TRX woman - mobile only conversions (6	Inactive	37 Leads	4,756	15,286	$6.30 Per Lead	$8.00 Daily	$233.26	Or
Copy 1 - group ab and pose - mobile only (convert L..	Inactive	66 Leads	7,411	21,530	$6.09 Per Lead	$8.00 Daily	$402.05	Or
Copy 1 - group pyramid pose - mobile only (switch t	Inactive	132 Leads	11,331	46,427	$5.85 Per Lead	$19.00 Daily	$772.46	Or
Results from 5 ad sets		281 Leads	14,710 People	94,805 Total	$5.56 Per Lead		$1,561.83 Total Spent	

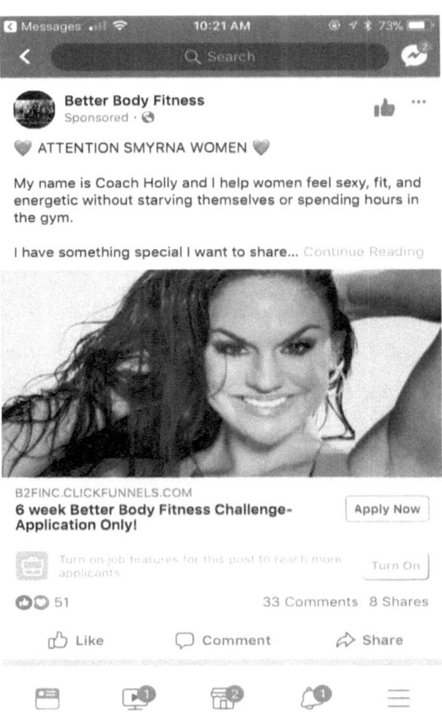

CHAPTER 5
DRIVE CONVERSIONS

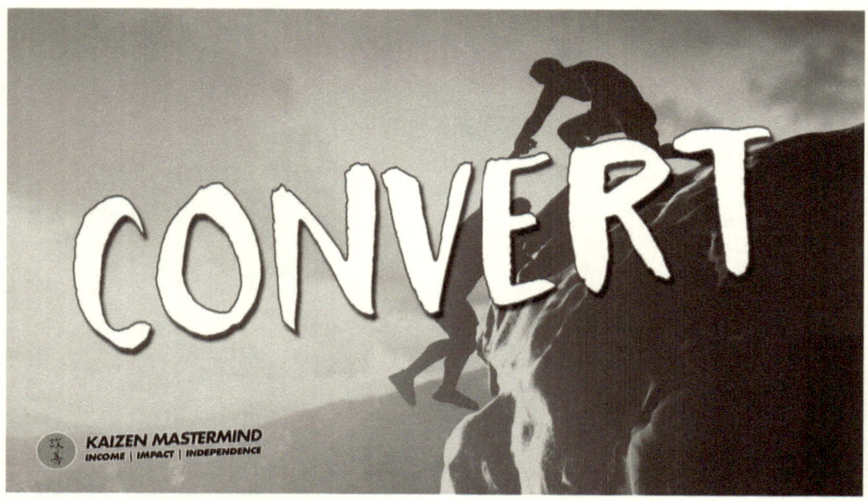

When someone says the word "conversion" to you, what comes to mind?

The truth is, it's an act of change. In the world of fitness, it's taking someone from where they are now to a much better future just by having them come along with you on this journey.

Conversions are not about the almighty dollar. The moment you place all of the value in making money instead of actually helping another person, you have just lost your client's long-term investment. The value comes in the process of converting them to your beliefs and values, and converting them to your tribe.

You're probably thinking that it sounds a little bit like a cult, right?

That can be a bit misleading. According to Russel Brunson, the author of many top-selling marketing books, "It's about creating a cult-ure." In other words, you are acting as their leader and superhero. Think back to Chapter 3: A.C.E, when we discussed that we're creating the authority, celebrity, and expert that people desire to follow.

The moment you understand and accept that you are playing a critical role in the market and that most people are looking for a leader is the moment that you will crush your competition by building a powerful following and making a real change in the world.

Of course, you must remember, it all starts with your client's *YES* to the sale.

Unfortunately, most trainers jump into the game and then wonder why they're not that great at selling. They start wondering why it's such a struggle to make people understand that they do have the solution to the problems keeping their prospects up at night. The challenge here is that most trainers believe that it's all about them. They don't think about interviewing their potential clients to gain an understanding of who they are, where they are going, or the challenges standing in their way.

Instead, they shine the light on themselves. They talk about how wonderful their program is or what a great trainer they are. After all, they have all the certifications to back it up, right? You must understand that no one really gives a shit about you—at least not at first. They want to see that you understand who they are and that you can empathize with them and their situation. Only then will they want to know if you have what it takes to get them past their roadblocks. Theodore Roosevelt, the 26th President of the United States said it best, "Nobody cares how much you know until they know how much you care."

As a trainer, what do you believe is the biggest challenge you are facing when it comes to selling?

COMMON CHALLENGES FOR TRAINERS

1. *They make it all about them.*

We just talked about this challenge, but it's the one that you really need to get a grasp on above the others. The number one challenge that trainers face is that they start with themselves and what makes them so special. The problem here is that it's too much about them. They center their pitch on "Look at me. Look at my service. Look at my body. I'm great. You need me to help you become like me."

Unfortunately, this is what many trainers actually believe. They don't seem to realize that this mindset keeps them from converting their prospects into clients. Many trainers simply think it should be all about them. Unless you want to be the person that is buying all the personal training yourself, then it's best to be focused on them and not you.

2. *They can't ask for the close.*

The second challenge that trainers face is asking for the close. It's a lot like going on a date and sitting on the couch with someone—what happens? You're sitting there, it's awkward, and you're confused. You keep thinking, "Should I? Shouldn't I?" It's been a great date, but if you can't make a move, you'll never know the outcome. You kill the "sale" by wishing them a good night and saying, *"Call me tomorrow."*

In the dating world, the close is that kiss at the end of the night. When it comes to selling, the close is asking the client for the sale. Too often, trainers put too much pressure on the close, and they can't ask for it because they're worried they'll be rejected. If you don't ask, they can't say no, right? You can get past all of that by simply saying:

"Mrs. Jones, would you like to get started today? I have two different offers for you, A or B. Which is the one that you believe would benefit you most?"

3. *They can't handle objections.*

The last problem that trainers face is that they can't handle objections. They're afraid of them. There are a handful of objections that people will give you in every selling situation, but trainers fear them like the plague. When it comes to asking for the close, you have the fear of rejection. However, when you get an objection, this is the point where you will feel like you're being rejected.

The funny thing is, that's just the story that you're telling yourself. The issue is that if you do get an objection, you just didn't dig deep enough to prove the true value of your program. You didn't force them to sit down with you and talk about your program. They came to you looking for answers, and objections are usually not the truth. You must keep in mind that they are nervous and uncertain, so you really can't fault them for saying things like:

"I have to talk it over with my spouse."

"That seems a little high right now for me."

"I have to think it over."

You should make it your goal to walk them through those objections instead of fighting them on it. If you can't handle objections, you just allowed someone who came to you with a problem walk right back out into that world of darkness. Then, they have to go searching for the next thing.

Which of these three challenges do you have the hardest time with?

At one time or another, you will have a challenge with one of the objections or even all of them, but over time you will build confidence with every prospect meeting you do. You want to get to the point where you develop bulletproof skin to handle objections that are thrown at you. That is when you know you have reached a level of mastery. And guess what? People are attracted to masters like magnets. With that being said, we'll share five mastery principles to get you there.

Create A Conversion Event

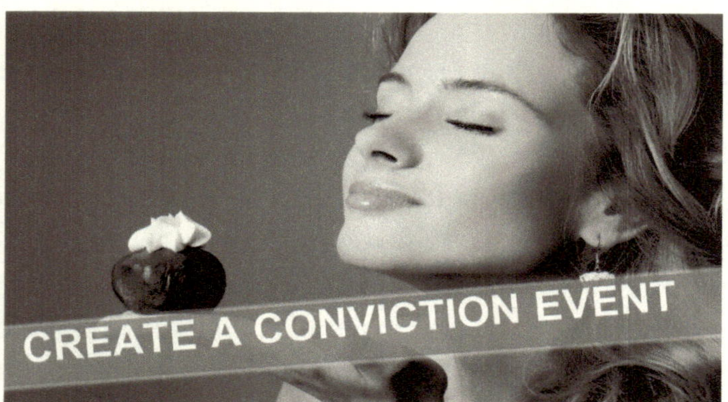

The very first mastery principle is that you must create a conversion event. What the hell is a conversion event? I'm so glad you asked! This is an offer/interaction that results in the prospect engaging with you. This can be anything at all from a free guide, a fitness challenge, a sample meal plan, a training session trial, sales page, webinars, direct messages on social media, etc. It must be something that causes your prospects to raise their hand to interact with you, creating a micro-commitment opportunity.

Three Buying Temperatures

The conversion event is about understanding the buying temperature of your prospect. Let's take a look at the three buying temperatures.

a. Hot: This is a lead that is ready. They've heard about you. They've been through your website. They've gone through your sales funnel. They are truly ready. They know you. They love you. They trust you. More than likely, these people are on your email list.

b. Warm: This is a lead that is not quite ready. They have seen you on social media. They may have even opted-in to your communications. However, they're not really ready to buy in. You need to spend some extra time convincing them.

c. Cold: This is a lead that hasn't heard of you and they don't even realize they need you. The only thing they know is they were surfing along just fine on social media and suddenly, your ad popped up. Cold leads are wondering, "Okay, who is this person, and what are they offering? Can I really trust them?"

Three Steps for a Successful Conversion Event

At this point, you must create a conversion event so that you can make sure to qualify them right away. These three things are necessary for a successful conversion event:

1. Create desire for your services/products.

2. Posture your offer.

3. Establish your authority on the situation.

Create Desire for Your Services/Products

Have you ever bought something from a company and asked what else they had because you liked it so much? Perhaps you liked the iPhone, which led you to desire another product from Apple like an iPad or an Apple Watch. Likewise, you want to go ahead and create the desire for your services and products for your clients. For example, you can create something for your audience like "The 7-Day Slim Down Meal Plan." Basically, it's a seven-day meal plan that your audience would receive by entering one of your funnels. After they get that, your audience might say, "Wow, I got these meal plans, what else does Meta Burn have to offer?"

Posture the Offer

Then we posture the offer. We are going to make sure that they know that we are the answer to their problem. Through our benefit copy, they can clearly see how the 7 Day Slim Down is exactly what they need. It's postured as being the BEST.

Establish Your Authority

Then we establish our authority by telling them what we specialize in and how we have helped over 1,000 women to date. They want to know others have been there before them and how their life has changed. Once these three things are in place, you have whet their appetite to walk through your sales funnel experience.

Conversion Qualifier

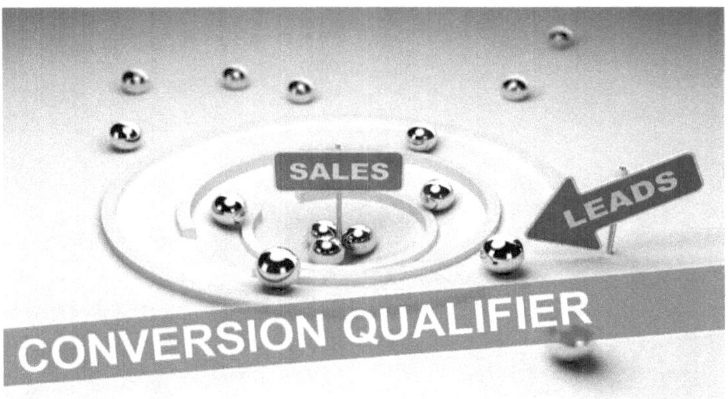

This brings us to the second principle which is a conversion qualifier. First, you have an "event." Then you have a qualifier to test their buying temperature like we mentioned above. This qualifier happens before you even speak to them.

This is the step that takes them from cold to warm and sometimes hot. Remember how we talked about micro-commitments in Chapter 4? Well, this is another step that increases that commitment because they are taking precious time out of their lives to continue the journey with you.

Once they opt-in to your front offer/event, now you are asking them to fill out an application, call you directly for a free bonus gift, buy this one time offer at a major discount to compliment the initial offer, or visit the studio for a tour.

If they take any of those actions, they are reconfirming their interest in what you have to offer and that they are in need of help. This helps you clear out the tire kickers because as professionals, we don't have time to waste on people that just want to suck the energy out of us.

Invisible Interview

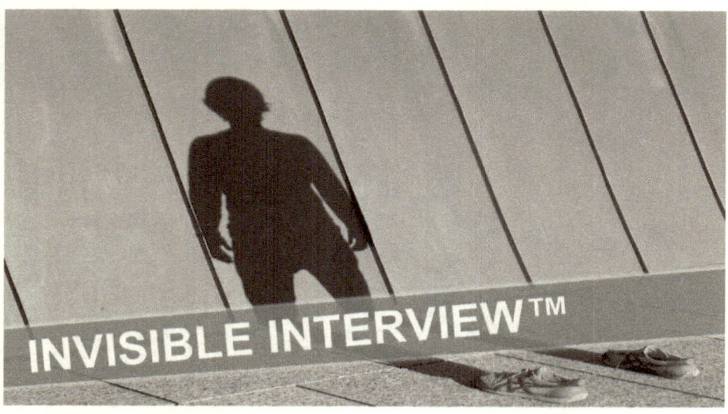

The third principle is literally a game changer: the invisible interview. We are always about optimizing our systems. Back in 2008 when we first opened the business, we didn't qualify anyone. If we placed a mirror under your nose and it fogged up, you were a perfect fit for our program. We accepted everyone. Come 2009, we realized that we were accepting people that weren't a great fit. So, we created a qualification call process, which worked very well for us, but it cost us a lot of time.

When a prospect raised their hand, we hopped on the phone and spend about 45-60 minutes trying to present why we were great, uncover their pain, and allow them to ask all the questions they had. We met some interesting people that could talk your ear off.

Out of necessity, we created the Invisible Interview. Our mentor Taki Moore back in 2015 was teaching the concept of interviewing a prospect versus being interviewed. He went over how he did that to us before we signed up, and a light bulb went off, like *Holy shit this really works*. So, we hashed out how this could work for our training business and came up with the name Invisible Interview because it was a process of questions, posturing, and directness that had the client interviewing for our programs without them even knowing it.

The Invisible Interview is an 11-minute interview script that will have your prospects begging you to become your client. It's another filter, but now it's live, and you are on the phone with the prospect asking them specific questions to test how serious they are and if they are a fit for your program and culture.

This cuts down your time drastically, and you can interview 20-30 people a day without feeling burned out. There are five steps within the Invisible Interview. In the worksheets you downloaded from **www.TheOneHourTrainer.com/worksheets**, we laid out those five steps of the Invisible Interview for you and the questions you ask.

At the end of the call, you decide if they are a fit or not. If they are, schedule a consultation. If not, let them go and try to point them in the right direction. When you follow this process, make sure to tell us how it changed your business; we know it will!

Smooth Outcome Session

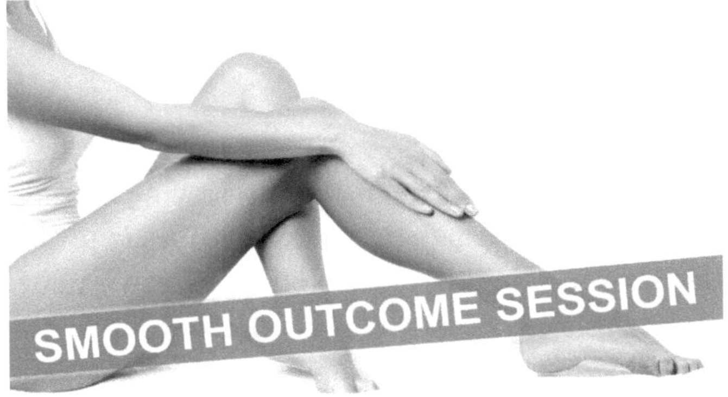

You've taken the time to filter your prospect through various processes to find out how committed they are. They've set up an appointment, and you're now going into the Smooth Outcome Session. Ultimately, you will get a firm "Yes" or a hesitant "No" because the value in your presentation wasn't high enough for them to object.

But we are going to make sure you deliver unbelievable value with our 7-step smooth outcome session. The reason we call it a smooth outcome session is because there are no bumps. Usually, there's no kickback. All there is to it is this: "Okay, that's great, fantastic. I'd love to do that." Then next thing you know, boom, they're a client.

Now, what are the seven steps to a smooth outcome session?

1. Create a Connection

2. Deep Dive

3. Check-in

4. Impact

5. Solution Reveal

6. Invite

7. Follow-up

This is called pull versus push. You're just laying it out for them, sharing why your solution is the answer to their problem, and letting the prospect make a decision. It doesn't matter what the decision is as long as they make a decision. You don't want wishy-washy people wasting your time, wasting your energy, and more importantly leading you down a rabbit hole where you're chasing them instead of them chasing you.

We are going to go into number one, creating that connection. Creating that connection is what we find a lot of personal trainers and newbies don't do very well. Remember, the problem with converting is that it's all about the trainer rather than the prospect. We want to make sure that you understand the key to this is making sure you create a connection. How do you create a connection within the first thirty seconds of a conversation or meeting your prospect? Look them in the eye, use their name, keep a smile, have confidence, and find something that you both can relate to.

Where do you live? How long have you lived in the area? What college did you go to? What's your favorite band? What's your favorite sports team? as long as you can build that connection and keep them engaged in an interesting conversation. You want them to know that you are not there to sell them, that you are there to listen.

Once you create some rapport, you can do a deep dive by asking more personal questions related to why they are sitting in front of you. For example, "Why us, why now? What made you pull the trigger to sit down with us now and not a few months ago?" or "How much weight do you want to lose? How long did it take you to put that weight on? What's been the impact that has had on your life?" The goal is to get them to open up and expose the pain they feel. Let's face it; no one is sitting there giddy and happy about making a change in their life.

Then, you check in so that you know that you're asking the right questions and you're leading them in the right direction within the sales process. You want to reiterate what they told you and ask them if that is correct. This solidifies you are listening and also shows you care because you want to customize the conversation around their needs.

Once you get the confirmation, it's time to open up the most emotional part which is the Impact. You want to ask them if they continue what they are doing, what impact will that have on their life? Sit back and let them tell you how bad things will be if they don't change, but you can't let them marinate in that.

Next, you have to flip it to the positive impact. For example, "Mrs. Jones, you just told me how bad it would be if you didn't change a thing. Let me ask you if we can help you accomplish XYZ in the next twelve weeks, how different would life be for you?"

They can then envision how happy they would be if you could help them get there. They are beginning to buy in because no one has ever helped them see the light at the end of the tunnel. To take it a step further, show them the impact it has had on clients that are just like them. Now you go into story mode of the impact of another client's journey.

This sets up the next step, which is the Solution Reveal. Now that they see the opportunity, it's time to lay out the plan and the solution. This is where you want to share exactly how your system works step by step, so they can see the roadmap. If you think just telling them you are going to work out for an hour three times a week is enough to entice them, you are going to lose a lot of people. You want to name your training system and how it operates, the philosophy and steps behind your nutrition approach, and how you have systems in place to keep them accountable and supported.

Once you draw them into the system and ask, "Does this all make sense? Can you see how this is not as hard as it seems and how we can turn things around?" Now it's time for the invite.

You are not selling them. You are simply stating that they would be a perfect fit for your program and inviting them into your house. This is where you say, "Mrs. Jones, it's obvious you are committed to making a change in your life, and you can see how our system can get you to your end goal, right? The last thing to go over is your options to work with us so we can see that smile on your face we just saw. We have X, Y, and Z programs. Based on what you told me, I would recommend Y and Z program. Which is the best fit for you?"

This is where you now…. SHUT UP!

Don't open your mouth. Don't backtrack. Don't say anything to interfere with their thought process.

You need to allow them to soak in this entire process because they are about to make a decision, or if the value wasn't high enough, give you an objection that is a false objection because they are nervous.

The last step is the follow-up. There are two scenarios.

If they said "Yes, I want to do this program," the follow-up is all about getting their credit card, cash, or check on the spot, have them fill out some basic paperwork, and reiterate how they will receive your program materials, how they can get in contact with you, and what the next step is in booking their first session.

If they presented an objection, that's usually a hesitant "No" which means now you need to follow-up with some questions on where things went wrong. Let's go through some examples of how to turn things around.

Objection #1: It's a bit out of my budget, and not sure I can afford it.

Your response: Thank you for being open with me, Mrs. Jones. We completely understand this is an investment and respect that. Just so I am understanding you, is it the total investment that is out of your budget, or if I were to break these down into X payments would that fit into your budget?

Outcome: This will tell you if it really is out of their budget or not because if they can't afford the payments, you don't want to be that trainer that pushes them by saying put it on a credit card and pay it off later. When you break it down, it makes it easier to swallow as a prospect, and most times they will say yes knowing there is a way you can work with them.

Objection #2: I have to think it over.

Your response: Your response: 100%. I know when I am about to buy something I like to think through everything, and there are usually some questions I have. You had mentioned that you really wanted to fit into that wedding dress and make it the best night of your life. I am just curious what is it that you need to think over so that I can help answer any questions you have while we are sitting together?

Outcome: This will usually open up questions to clarify this is the best program for them or will open up the underlying objection which could be finances or that they are not the primary buyer in the household, which you can handle separately.

Objection #3: I need to talk it over with my spouse

Your response: Absolutely, I know that when I make an investment in something I like to involve my spouse in the process so there is no misunderstanding. What do you think your spouse would say about you joining this program today? Ok, great, is there a time we can set up an appointment with your spouse so I can share with them the value of this program for you?

Outcome: Have them open up if they are the primary buyer or if finances really need to be discussed due to their situation. If they are not the primary buyer, the goal is to see how you can show the primary buyer the same value you just showed them.

That's the simple 7-step process of converting prospects into clients. But there is one more step!

Celebrate Their Victory

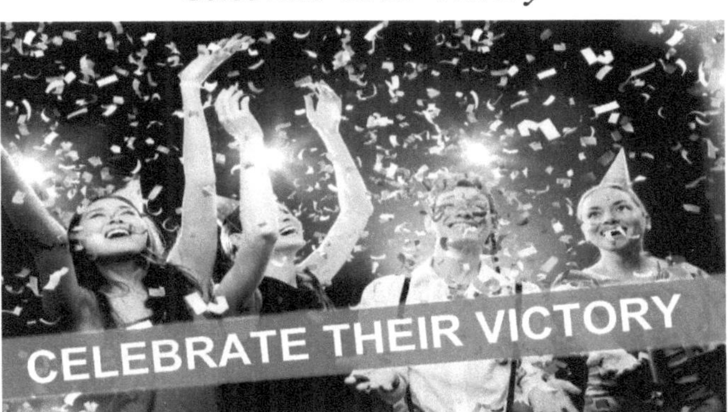

This is crucial! Most times, trainers miss this when they collect the money. Miss this principle, and it's kind of like accomplishing a goal that you were so excited for and when you share it with someone, you can tell they couldn't care less and don't join in on that excitement.

It's like feeling left out or like what you did wasn't good enough. When a prospect hands over their hard-earned money, they want you to celebrate with them on their victory for making a change.

You can't dismiss this, or buyer's remorse kicks in.

Upon getting payment, you want to tell them how excited you are to have them join the family and how you can't wait to see their transformation from X days from now. Reiterate that this is a decision that will change their life.

With that, make sure they leave with something. We recommend a folder with information about you and a welcome letter along with a free gift for them to take home.

There is a whole onboarding process you want to take, which is outside the scope of this book, but here is the piece they need to leave with and what we do at Meta Burn Fitness as their celebration.

We hand them a red folder with a welcome letter, referral letter and card, supplement checklist, and a flyer that gives them reading material on what Meta Burn stands for and how they get great results. To top it off, they receive a welcome box with another letter expressing our excitement, an aluminum branded water bottle, a branded sweat towel for their workouts, and a branded journal to log notes of their journey.

To seal the relationship even tighter, within an hour, they receive a welcome email with all the nutrition materials from our nutrition director. As a follow-up to that email, there is a text from our nutrition director personally welcoming them, alerting them that their materials were just sent, and setting up a time for the nutrition kick-off call to walk them through the program.

All of this is done to celebrate their victory of coming on board with us, and along the way, we recognize their accomplishments. These celebration steps cost around $15 and 15-20 minutes of your time to tie the bond.

Now that you know the five mastery principles behind driving conversions, which one of the five would have the greatest impact on your sales? Circle one below and get to work:

a) Creating a conversion event

b) Producing a conversion qualifier

c) Implementing an invisible interview

d) Operating a smooth outcome session

e) Celebrating the victory

You must commit to attracting your clients with a relaxed selling process. If you're committed to that, we can promise you that this business will be so much easier for you. You will create a lifestyle fitness business that you will love and stands out from the competition. More sales made equals more lives changed. Commit to changing more lives, and your life will enhance along the way.

Want to upgrade your sales process and start charging premium prices for your valuable services? Check out **www.BlackBeltSellingMethod.com/onehour** *for a special discount as our appreciation for picking up a copy of this book and committing to create a One Hour Trainer lifestyle.*

Chapter 6
CREATE RAVING FANS

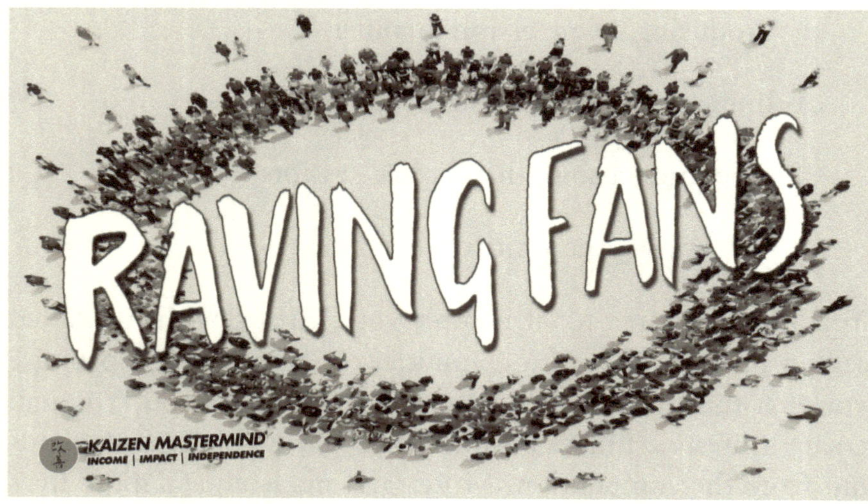

Do you remember a moment in your life where you had your mom or dad, or perhaps your dear friends, cheering you on from the crowd? Maybe it was a sports match, a graduation or some kind of competition. Whether something happened negatively or not they were there to cheer you on and helped show their support for you.

This is a core strategy for developing a world-class fitness business. Not only for the growth of the company but also predictability and consistency. Your clients are the bedrock of a solid business. Treat them right, and they will hold you up. Treat them wrong, and they will erode quickly and your business will crumble.

They are the ones that will lead you to more referrals and more business than any other spoke on your marketing wheel. So, why do trainers spend more time hunting for prospects than focusing on their current business? That's what this chapter will reveal to you: how you will be able to break through the monotony and understand the five mastery principles to creating raving fans.

Let me share a story from our business to give you some context to exactly what this means to a business.

Lorraine A. is one of our outstanding clients that came from a typical Facebook ad. She came in, sat down for the consultation, and was closed immediately on a 12-week transformation, a $1,000 program. Not a bad sale for someone who has never heard of you and just clicked on your ad. What will shock you is that $1,000 sale alone actually generated us $55,847 within a 3-year period of time that didn't cost us a cent in advertising. Lorraine had begun referring her friends to us within 3 weeks due to the amazing results and experience she received. Now, not all clients will be a raving fan like Lorraine, but when you follow this chapter, you will see the power that a raving fan can have for your business.

How were we able to generate an additional $55,847 from Lorraine?

We have an onboarding process that indoctrinates every new client into creating them into a raving fan. But more importantly, we are a results-based company, and we focus on the client, not on ourselves. So, within the first 30 days (and of course it doesn't stop), we really are honing in on making sure that they're happy, that they feel comfortable, and that there's 100% clarity in what we're asking of them and what they can expect of us. This led to Lorraine introducing her best friend to the program. Christine came in, crushed the program, lost 17 pounds in 6 weeks, and the rest is history.

They live in a small town called Bayville. Woman after woman started coming in and signing up. We ended up with 14 new clients, $55,847 in revenue, and at the writing of this book, we still have clients active from Lorraine three years ago. Even after her best friend, Christine, stopped training with us, she still credits us as changing her life. She highlights us as the best personal training and nutrition coaching company for women in the area. She's come to tons of other events that we host. She's still a part of our community. She still participates in our private Facebook group. And this is all because we understand that once you create one raving fan, your business can explode without having to spend a ton of money on marketing. It can cost you nothing to double the size of your business.

More customers are going to come because they trust their friends, and referrals are the best way to build a lifestyle fitness business because it cuts down on how much money you have to invest in marketing. Once you get one fan, one should equal three to four new clients. Being in the service business, do not overlook the value of creating raving fans; it's powerful. I have a question for you. What business are you in? What business are you really in? I want you to think about that, because you might have thought, *I'm in the personal training business, I'm in the nutrition business, I'm in the coaching business,* or *I'm in the boot camp business.*

You are not in any of those businesses. The business that you're really in is the service business. The service business is a business where you serve people and help them create the best versions of themselves. It's not about counting reps or showing up to cheer them on. You are there to serve above and beyond.

When you do this, your clients will return the favor, give you their contacts, and refer people to you. They speak about you. They become part of your culture and your tribe. This entire chapter is designed to help you do exactly what we did, how we attracted Lorraine and then how she helped us get new clients over and over again. But this is the great part: once you automate this process, it's going to put your business on steroids.

It's been a game changer for our business. Now, we have a process for every time we bring a new prospect to a client, from a client to a raving fan. We know how long it takes, and most importantly, that's our number one focus on delivering the BOOM to those new clients. It is crucial for your business.

It's clear that this stuff flat out works, leading us to ask the question, Why aren't more personal trainers doing this? Many personal trainers aren't currently creating raving fans because it's time-consuming. It takes a lot of time to actually make sure that each of your new clients come on board and is excited about your program, know exactly what to do, when to do it, how to do it, and know exactly how to refer to you properly.

This is why knowing your unique selling proposition is so important. Many new businesses that are just starting out—and even more seasoned businesses—miss this. It's one of the first things that we make sure we explain clearly to our new clients so that they know how to articulate specifically what it is we do, why we're unique, and why we're the best in the industry for what we do. Our unique selling proposition is we are the best personal training and nutrition coaching team for the greater Long Island area, specifically helping women overcome pre and post-menopausal weight loss challenges. When they tell their friends that, especially if they're in the age of 40 to 60, they want to work with Meta Burn Fitness.

We want you to understand that the time-consuming part of it is just setting up a system, automating that system, utilizing your team, and most importantly, making sure that you inspect what you expect, making sure that your team is pushing the process through properly.

The second problem is that it's tedious. You do have to put work into this. You have to tweak it. You have to test it. You have to redo it over and over again because you want to make sure that you're always improving, right? You have to have a Kaizen mindset, constantly and always improving. And as long as you're constantly and always improving, you're going to be able to create raving fans.

The third thing is sometimes the process must be manual. It's just the way it is. If you want to do it effectively, do not always rely on software and machines, not everything should be automated. There are some things that you have to touch in order to make them work.

The main fear around creating a raving fan culture from our conversations with trainers is that it's going to increase their amount of workload outside of the session. But what I can promise you is that more work on your current clients is a blessing because you don't always want to be on the hunt finding new people and hoping that Facebook, Instagram, Google, or any other platform is just going to send you leads with ease.

This is a simple process that you can install in your business and start winning right away. You want to streamline this process so that it's fun and enjoyable, then automate it so that it's effective and efficient. The ultimate aspiration for any business owner is to reap an amazing number of new referrals, keep their clients longer, and most importantly, plant the seed so that you can do it over and over again and make it work for you, just like we did with Lorraine, Christine, and her friends.

Here are the five mastery principles behind creating raving fans:

Amazing On-Boarding Experience

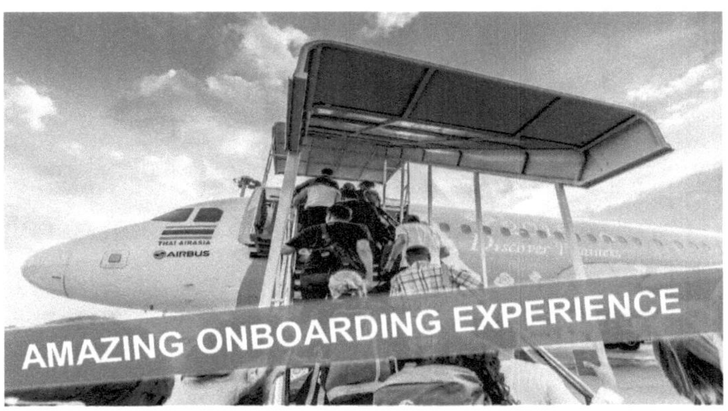

Imagine if getting on a plane was the opposite of what it is now. Imagine there was no system for on-boarding. As soon as the plane lands the passengers get off and everyone waiting to go on the next flight just rushes on. No checking bags, no scanning tickets, no system for seating, passengers can sit anywhere, the plane wasn't cleaned because everyone rushed on, and there were no signs on board to tell you what to do. Imagine people smoking cigarettes, talking on their cell phones, and taking up extra seats because they don't want anyone sitting next to them.

Would you want to get on that plane? I wouldn't. That's a miserable experience. Flying is not pleasant at times as it is, but you can imagine the chaos without an onboarding process.

We already touched upon this in detail in Chapter 5, so I don't want to beat a dead horse, but to summarize, upon a client signing up, they get a red folder that we walk them through. Inside is how to contact us, a welcome letter, the referral program, and a heavy graphic flyer on what Meta Burn is all about. They also leave with what we call our swag box with a branded water bottle, a sweat towel, journal, and thank you card.

Next, they receive next a welcome email with nutrition materials, a scheduled nutrition kick-off call to walk them through the program, access to our private Meta Burn app, and introduction to the Meta Burn family in our private Facebook group.

Over the next thirty days, we have several touch points via text message and calls, making sure that the new client knows exactly where they're going and how we're going to help them get there. They get a fitness assessment as their first session and weekly weigh-ins and body fat testing. Our coaches have a protocol of questions they ask each session to ensure the experience is top notch.

Our studios are kept clean daily, we provide fresh towels, and the culture of the gym is very friendly, supportive, and respectful.

Compared to big box gyms or local competitors that often just focus on working out a client, you can see how our on-boarding experience sets the tone for each new client and sets us also apart from the competition.

High Touch

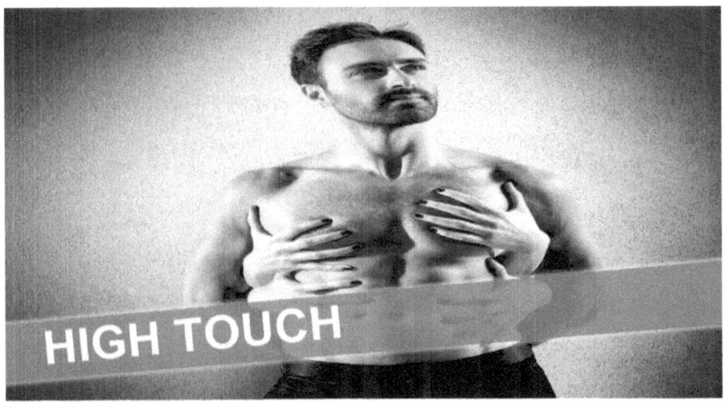

Principle number two is high touch. You want to make sure that you have a personal feel to your business. What do we do that adds that personal feel? One, we send out birthday cards that are handwritten with a $5 Starbucks card to every client who has a birthday. Now, you're probably wondering, "*Coach Rahz, five dollars? What is that?*" It's not the amount that matters, it's the thought that counts. So why do we use this? Because we get so many people that say, "*Thank you so much for my Starbucks card. I am so excited. I used it today.*" I want them to be consistently thinking about us. It helps us achieve TOMA, top of the mind awareness.

When you have your clients and customers out in the world thinking about you, what are they going to do? They're going to tell people. When they're using your towel and doing cardio outside of your studio, what are they going to do? Tell people where they got it. Your water bottle, too. These are all things that you should have as part of your high touch approach.

Then, we do something in our private group called check-in Fridays. We put up a post and ask, "What are your wins this week?" We want to highlight their wins. With every person who checks-in the comment box, a member of our staff makes sure to leave a response.

«Awesome job, Sally. You crushed your workout today. Fantastic.» This is high touch. You can automate it, but it must be personal.

We also use a google text line and private Meta Burn app just to check in and see how their week is going or what their next goal is for the week. All staff members (coaches, directors, nutrition coaches, admins, and owners) touch in at some point, so clients feel the love from all angles.

Culture

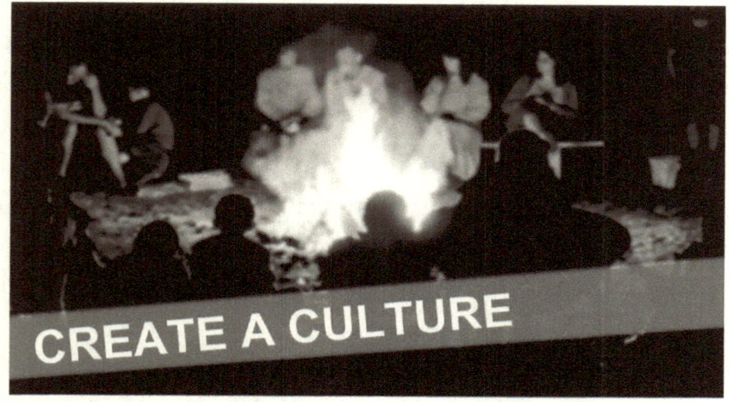

Mastery principle number three is culture. How are you creating your culture? How are you cultivating your tribe? One of the ways we do it is through language. We say, *"Hey, you're part of the Meta Burn family."* We start talking about the Meta Burn family right at the point of sale. We plant the seed that they are part of a family.

They're not just joining some gym. They're not joining a studio. They're not joining a fat loss program. They're joining a family. The word family connects support, love, and safety.

We also have client ambassadors. We select several different client ambassadors. Why do we do this? Because we want them out there raising their hands. We know that men die for it and babies cry for it; it's called recognition. When people get recognized as being selected, special, or exclusive, it heightens their feeling of significance. Ambassadors represent the brand, and they keep all clients connected.

We host several free workshops for clients throughout the year and also host gatherings like potlucks, barbecues, wine and cheese support nights, and other events to keep us connected.

We use certain language and gestures that all clients adapt and start using. For instance, we use the words BOOM, rock star, superstar, crush it, let's burn, and other phrases we found our women love hearing and saying. We also end every single session with a high five. No matter what, that is mandatory for each coach to initiate. Clients will literally wait until they get a high five before they leave.

What are three things you can implement over the next four weeks to improve your culture?

Reward Your Best Clients

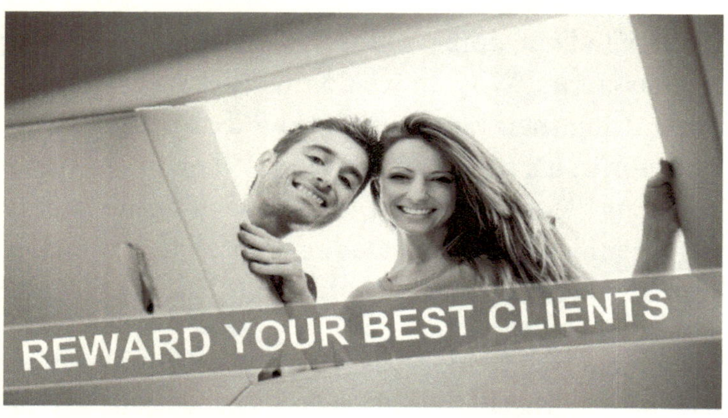

Principle number four is rewarding your best clients. This is where technology is helpful. You can use whatever software to track the amount of revenue clients are bringing in, referrals or amount of sessions used, and results. You want to know the metrics on your clients.

So yes, we treat everybody amazing. They're all part of that family. But it's smart to set up recognition milestones so everyone has something to shoot for. If they are big spenders, we will send a gift like a free massage. If they refer their friends, we give them free sessions. If they use a certain amount of sessions, we will recognize them publicly for being committed. If they rock out their results and have the best ones of the month, they will be publicly recognized as the client of the month, and we will send them a $5 Starbucks gift card.

You can take it a step further and customize gifts based on your client's interests. That will take some time to develop notes during sessions or stalking them on social media.

What we want you to understand as the fitness entrepreneur creating a fitness lifestyle business is that you don't want to have pennies in your eyes on your way to millions. You want to be able to see through the forest, see the light at the end of the tunnel, and understand that what we're sharing with you in this book will change your business because it has for us.

We want you to pick one client in the next 24 hours that you can publicly recognize for an accomplishment ,and we want you to send them a hand-written note with a $5 Starbucks or Amazon gift card.

Surveying Your Clients

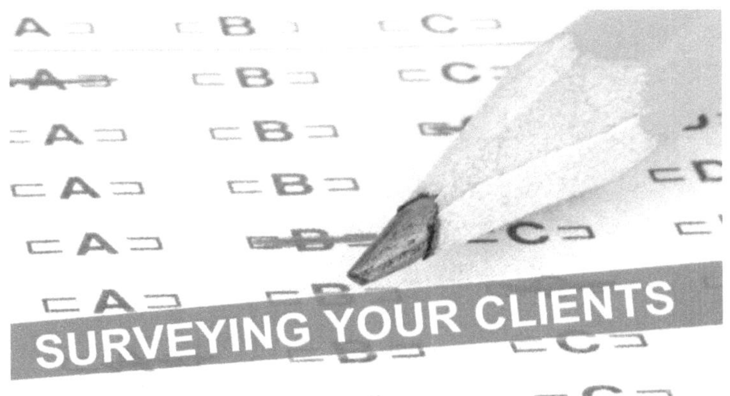

If you are going to reward them, you might as well survey them. Mastery principle number five is surveying your clients, and this one is going to take some work as well but is well worth it. Surveys help you know what's working, what's not working, and feedback on how to improve your program, environment, and experience.

Make this anonymous using Wufoo Forms or Survey Monkey. Take your ego and feelings out of the equation, and just read the words on each survey as the current facts of your client's current perceptions.

When was the last time you surveyed your entire client list to hear what they have to say about their experience? And I'm talking buyers, people who pay you money currently. When was it?

Was it the last 30 days? 60 days? 90 days? You should be doing this every 90 days, finding out what's working and what's not working in your organization, because I want you to have a Kaizen mindset, constantly and always improving. The only way you're going to do that is by getting feedback and using the feedback loop in order to tweak the things you need to change and improve your business. This allows you to have constant growth and help you innovate faster than anyone who is trying to imitate you.

A great method to get feedback from inactive clients is only emailing them with a one to three sentence email. "Hey, just checking in. Can you help me out? Why did you stop training at XYZ gym?" That's a great one.

A third method is you can have an exit survey they fill out. Every time a client leaves, you want to make sure you get their feedback but also give yourself another opportunity to pull them back in. In our business, we pull back in one out of every ten clients that leave, and we have a nine-month retention rate, whether they come in on a six-week or a twelve-week program.

So out of those five mastery principles, which one can you focus on in the next week? Is it number one, creating an onboarding experience that is just lights out, world-class? Can you add in a little bit more high touch personal feeling in your creating raving fans system? What is one thing that you can do to start to create and embed a culture in your clients and in your environment? How can you reward your clients? Are you surveying them so that you know exactly what they want, when they want it, and how you can deliver it to them?

We want you to create a world-class fitness facility that will create a lifestyle for you and your family so that you can have more income, create more impact, and live with more independence. Tony Robbins said it this way when we went to his 6-Day Business Mastery program, "The biggest mistake organizations make is that they fall in love with their business or product and not their clients." We don't want you to make that mistake. We want you to fall in love with your clients. It is crucial for your business. It's crucial for you to grow and scale. If you fall in love with your clients, they're going to fall in love with you and help you reach the One Hour Trainer lifestyle.

PART 3: SYSTEMIZE

Chapter 7
ANAZLYZE TRACKING

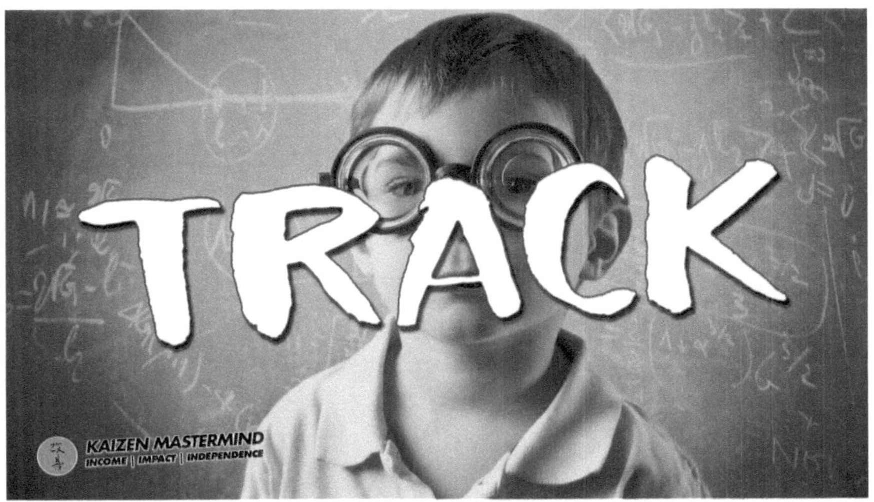

You have a doctor's appointment you know you need to attend and probably should have done it months ago, but you kept putting it off. As important as it is that you go, you already have a point of reference of what to expect.

Upon showing up five minutes early for your visit, you notice that the doctor's office is filled with patients before you so that's your signal for you to sit your ass down and wait an hour until they catch up.

Fine, you don't mind a little wait, but then they slapped you with papers you already filled out at your last doctor visit, and they keep asking you the same shit as if your social, name, date of birth, or care of HIPPA policy has changed. To add insult to injury, they don't make you fill that out so the doctor can look it over; it's just for your file. When it's time to see the doctor, he's going to ask you the same questions that you already filled out.

Now that you know you have some time to kill before it's your turn, you grab a magazine and flip through it 2-3 times pretending to read it. You just need some type of visual stimulation. What feels like hours of reading was only five minutes according to your phone. Instead of going back to the magazine, you open your phone and start texting people, scrolling Facebook, Instagram, or Snapchat, or reading your email. But the moment you realize there's nothing exciting, you continue to flip through each app just in case something has changed from a second ago or maybe someone thought of you to reach out, only to discover that nothing has changed, and you feel like your life is wasting away, but it's still important you went because once you see the doctor, he tells you, "It's great you came in today because if you waited any longer, it would have been much worse."

That's exactly what tracking numbers feels like to trainers. It's fucking boring and overwhelming at times, and you end up making emotional decisions because you don't have time to be logical. It's kind of like being trapped under a sheet of ice gasping for air.

We hate numbers and tracking just as much as you do, but it's the difference between thriving versus dying.

Our hope is this chapter shows you how to simplify the process, be strategic about your decisions, and open up opportunities so you can be on the move and grow your business.

What are you currently tracking in your business?

Here are the five principles you want to know whether you are solo or have a team. This will be short and sweet so we can move on to other fun parts of being a Lifestyle Fitness Business.

Marketing

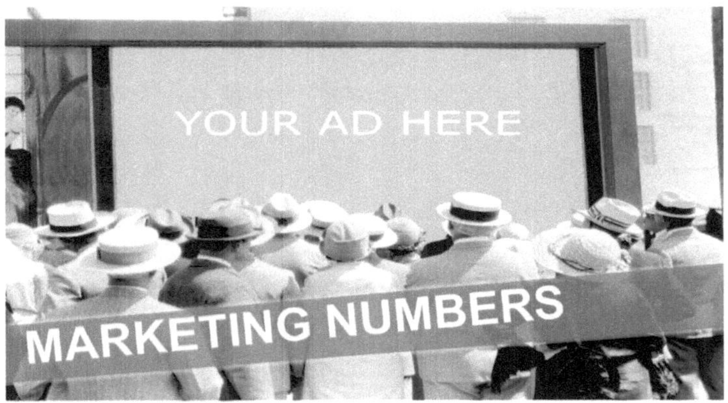

When marketing to attract new clients, whether its online or offline media, you want to separate each piece into a campaign, so you know the total costs and total revenue from that campaign.

Let's use Facebook advertising as an example. Let's say I have a 12 Week Challenge I am running, and I set up an ad to fill that program. There are only three important numbers you need to know from this.

1. *How much did the ad campaign cost me in total?*

2. *What was my cost per lead?*

3. *What was the cost to acquire a new client?*

Let's say you ran an ad and spent $1,000 total. From that campaign, you generated 100 leads. 100 people gave you their name, email, and number to talk about the program. From those 100 leads, 25 people actually gave you money for your program.

How much did the ad campaign cost in total? $1,000

What was my cost per lead? $1,000 cost divided by 100 leads = $10

What was the cost to acquire a new client? 100 leads divided by 25 bought times $10 cost per lead = $40 to acquire new client

It's not fun to do this, but it's very important because if it costs you, for example, $200 to get a new client and you are selling them a $1,000 12-week challenge, you get all excited thinking you just made $1,000 but actually only made $800 before any additional expenses. You may be saying "Duh, I knew that," but for every one trainer that does, nine others have no clue.

Finance

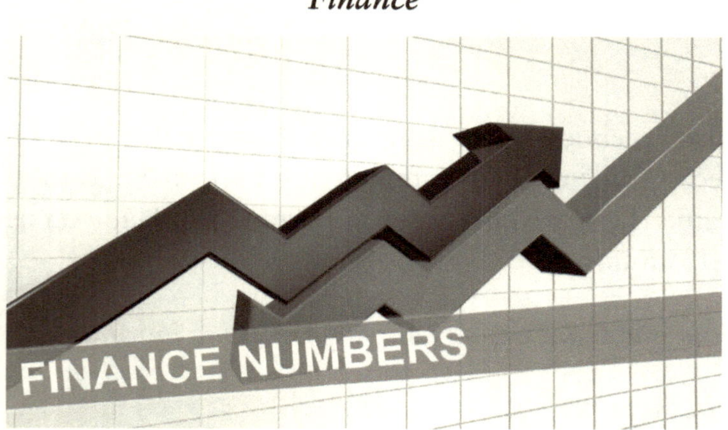

Ever take a finance or accounting class in college? They teach you shit you'll never use again. The three important things you need to know in the finance pillar is

1. Monthly Revenue

2. Monthly Expenses

3. Net Profit

It's that simple, but do you know what those three numbers were from last month? Were you in a profit or loss for that month? Most trainers don't take the time to track these things. They see they made $10,000 for the month, took home $5,000 in their pocket as profits, and charge $5,000 on the credit card for a new machine or coaching program because they have $5,000 left over. What they forget is they had a monthly expense of $3,000 to cover rent, utilities, gas, taxes, insurance, and possibly payroll if they have a team.

Now they are negative $3,000, and when they realize when it's time to pay the credit card bill that they don't have the money.

You may be shaking your head and saying, "What an idiot," but have you ever wondered where the money went in your business and how come your account is so low you can't pay off your bills?

It happens to more trainers than you can imagine because they focus only on monthly revenue and wing their expenses and profits.

Simple software like QuickBooks can track all of this for you.

Sales

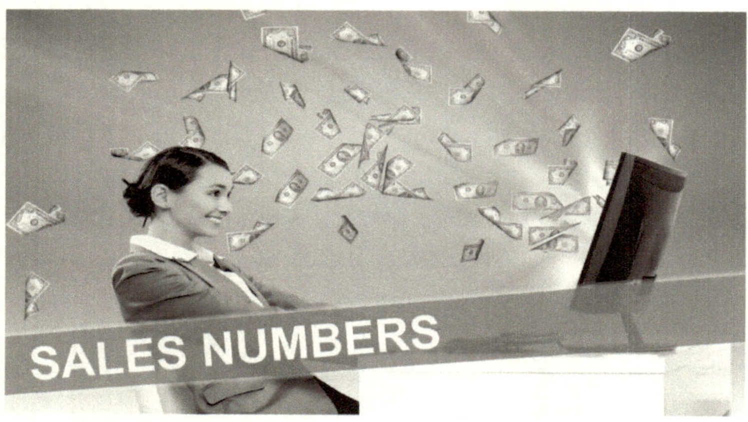

Bored yet? Stick with us because this will prevent you from going broke and allow you to thrive in this industry.

There are 3 categories to track in sales.

1. Set, Show, Close

2. Monthly NEW Sales

3. EFT (Electronic Funds Transfer)

The Set, Show, Close method is the easiest way to track your conversion rates and the pace your business is growing. What it simply means is how many appointments/consults have you Set for the week? Of those appointments, how many Showed, and finally from those who showed, how many were Closed?

We will break down what each component means to your business and how to optimize them.

SET – This is the component that will tell you if you are doing just busy work or productive work. If you are just keeping busy and not putting yourself out there, your set numbers will be really low if not zero. This component gives you an idea of how many people are actually interested in your program.

If your set number is low, the way to optimize it is by marketing harder. Whether it's setting up Facebook ads and spending money, asking clients for referrals, doing lunch and learn workshops, etc. You need to be putting yourself out there either in the belly to belly world or on social media with calls to action.

SHOW – This is the component that will tell you either how many people are really interested in your program or how well you are following up to confirm the appointment. You have to remember that people are busy and forget things easily. It doesn't matter how excited they sound on an initial call; you are not their #1 priority.

If your show number is low, the way to optimize it is by reiterating the date, time, and address on your initial set call, and either the night before or the morning of texting or calling them saying how excited you are to meet them at XYZ time on the set date. Most times people forget, and some are just not interested anymore. By following up, you increase your sales potential and get rid of any tire kickers that will waste your time.

CLOSE – This is the component that will tell you how good you are at sales and your conversion rate. You set the appointments. A percentage of them showed up, and now it's time to put your magic in place to close them to drive your sales.

If your close number is low, you need to get better at sales if you are going to survive in this business. We know you came into this to change lives, but if you don't focus on becoming better at sales, you no longer have the opportunity to change lives. There are only two options at every consult: either you sell them on why your program is the best thing for them, or they sell you on why it's not the right fit.

Track these numbers weekly and monthly so you can see patterns and be able to predict cash flow.

Monthly new sales are crucial to track because it shows your growth. There's going to be a time in your business if it hasn't already where a chunk of clients seemed to have had a conversation and all quit at the same time. It makes a huge dent in your business, and because you were focusing on how well things were going with your current clients, you took your eye off acquiring new ones. Trust us, you want new sales coming in each month because this business can be a roller coaster at times.

The last category is your EFT (electronic funds transfer), which is the money you can count on each and every month based on your client's contract. If you don't have recurring revenue in your business, you are making a mistake. On the 3rd of every month, based on which program we are launching, we cover 1/3-1/2 our monthly revenue goal without having to work for it. The system just charges the card on file. We love high ticket programs, but we also love to balance that out with monthly EFT charges.

Sales fix everything, so if you aren't tracking it, most likely you will be scratching your head as to why your bank account is so low.

Management

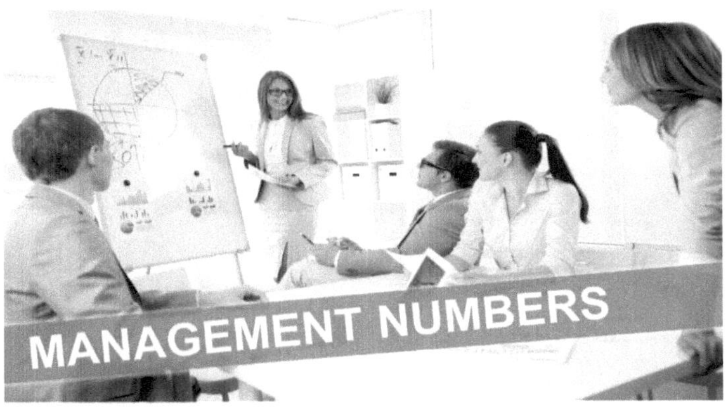

You can drive yourself crazy or you can simplify things. There's really only three things to track from the management side. They are:

1. Payroll

2. Total Client Sessions Trained

3. Staff Performance

Whether you are solo or you have a team, payroll is something you want to keep track of. It's the total amount you pay yourself and your team. We highly suggest you outsource your payroll to a professional so the right amount of taxes is taken out properly and you or your staff does not have to worry about a large chunk of taxes being taken out at the end of the year. Payroll taxes are one of those things you don't want to play games with due to the heavy fines and fees if anything is caught being done wrong. We are not telling you what to do with the cash under your mattress, but anything collected via check or credit card, it's better to claim on your payroll.

You have services like ADP that can work with small businesses and make sure all paperwork and tax work is in order.

The reason why you want to track your payroll and look at your numbers is so you can predict what you are feeding you and your team and what you are feeding your business. If you are extracting every single profit from the business, it's going to starve and face some very difficult times.

We are not financial advisors—nor are we giving professional advice—but the way we have successfully built our businesses is feeding the business first and taking the bare minimum we can survive on. This helps you pay your staff, invest in the business, and make improvements.

Total client sessions trained is crucial because each month you want to be able to track your growth or decline. This gives you patterns for the year as to what each month has produced as well as a way to set goals for the following year based on those numbers. Trainers typically don't track sessions very well, or if they do,, they use a spread sheet for clients when they run out of sessions, but they have no idea how many sessions the business did that month or that year. That's why we highly suggest using a client management software to do all of this for you, and you can run reports instantly. Software like Mindbody or Zenplanner are great (there are plenty more, so do your research).

Staff performance is not only great to know how the company is doing as a whole but also to recognize your staff, reward them, and help them set up new goals based on their previous performance to help them grow. This is easily done through a client management software.

Overlooking your management numbers stated above are just the top three things to track. Can you track more numbers? Sure, but it only makes business way more complex. When you hit $500,000 you can invest in more ways to track other data, but for now, keep it simple.

Customer Service

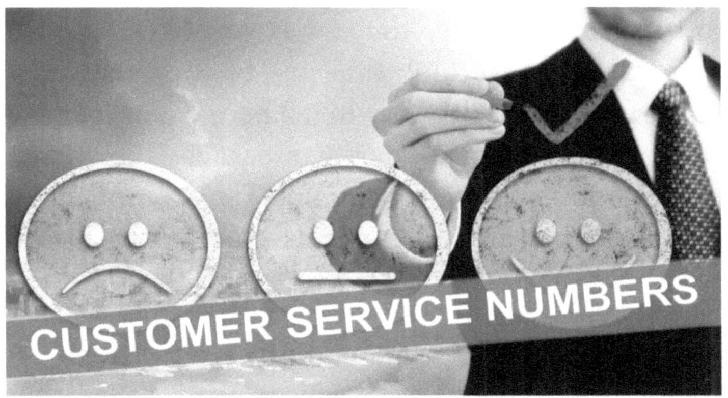

Keep those eyes open, because we are almost at the end of Tracking. The top three Customer Service numbers to track are:

1. Active Clients

2. Client's Lost

3. FEO Conversions

It sounds like a no-brainer to track your active clients, but we can't tell you how many times trainers have filled out a survey and said they don't know how many active clients they have. They have to go count. Again, a client management software can track that and pull it within seconds. It's easy to think you have more clients than actually present. Knowing how many are active helps you estimate your monthly income as well as using as a benchmark to reach your max capacity. Once you set the max capacity you and your business can handle, you now have a goal to shoot for.

Regardless of how great your business is, there will ALWAYS be clients that are going to leave; that's just how it is. Tracking clients lost is just as important. Tracking the number of clients that leave each month will give you some idea as to what you can expect the next month as well as knowing how many you need to bring in to replace those that you have lost. Unfortunately, trainers tend to think that just because they're making sales that their business is growing. Then, when they stop and take a look at their finances, they wonder why they're not making as much money as they thought. They're not making the money because they are losing clients—and we try not to think too hard about that.

What we mean by FEO is front-end offer conversions. No matter how a prospect became a new client, that's called your front end. It can be a low barrier offer, or it can be a high-end 12-week challenge. Either way, those are being tracked in your monthly new sales. Here, you want to focus on retention and how many of those FEO's convert over to ongoing clients. It's great to make a sale, but it's more powerful to growing the company to keep that person buying into your services. It's harder to acquire a brand-new client than it is to keep current ones happy.

You've reached the end of the tracking chapter. We understand this is not fun, but if you don't know your numbers, you are leaving yourself open and vulnerable to a disaster to strike. Even if you have a professional bookkeeper or accountant, you still need to know your numbers because there are certain things they won't track for you. Look at the ***Magic 15 KPI Tracker*** worksheet, keep it on your desk for the next few months, and start tracking those fifteen categories.

Chapter 8
DESIGN OPERATING SYSTEMS

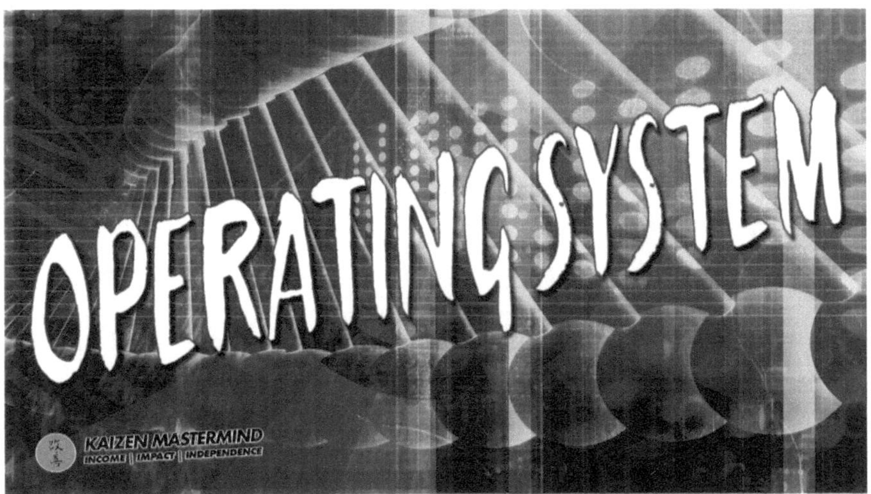

Are you a Mac or PC fan?

No judgment. We know it can be a heated battle between consumers on which is better. We use both within our businesses and don't have any issues with either.

Let's discuss the most important part of these computers. What runs both of them?

Before any newly manufactured computer (Mac or PC) can be used, an operating system (OS) needs to be installed on it. All the components in the operating system serve to make the various parts of a computer function in synergy. Synergy is the key.

We have been talking over the last seven chapters on how to create the One Hour Trainer lifestyle fitness business. In the space of business consulting, all you hear about is systems, systems, systems. But most times, consultants make things very complicated for personal trainers by having them install systems that do not make sense for them in their current situation. Because they look cool in theory or drawing them on a whiteboard, it's enticing for a personal trainer to want to jump on board to improve his/her business.

But we are here to tell you that you only want to install the systems that are going to make your life better, that are easy to operate not only by you, but also your team members, and don't handcuff you or make it really expensive to change.

Unfortunately, a lot of personal trainers, coaches, and business owners are currently on what we call the roller coaster model. That is, they are trying to tame the chaos in their business, and the reason they're struggling is that they don't know what systems they need in place to grow and scale their business. In addition, they're trying to do everything manually. When you try to build your business manually, you'll discover that there will be times when things will break down and you become a professional firefighter always putting fires out in the business. How you deal with those fires will determine whether your business will be successful or crash and burn.

We will be perfectly honest with you. When we started Meta Burn Fitness, we were a jack of all trades and a master of none. We did all five major pillars: sales, marketing, operations, customer service, and financials. We learned exactly how to do those things, and we did them manually without ever creating a system for each task. However, what we also learned in Michael Gerber's book, "The E-Myth" is that you can't grow your business to the next level if you're wearing all of the hats and carrying all the bricks.

You must understand that there will come a time when you will need to automate processes and systemize your business so that it will run smoothly. As a side note, I've never met or heard of

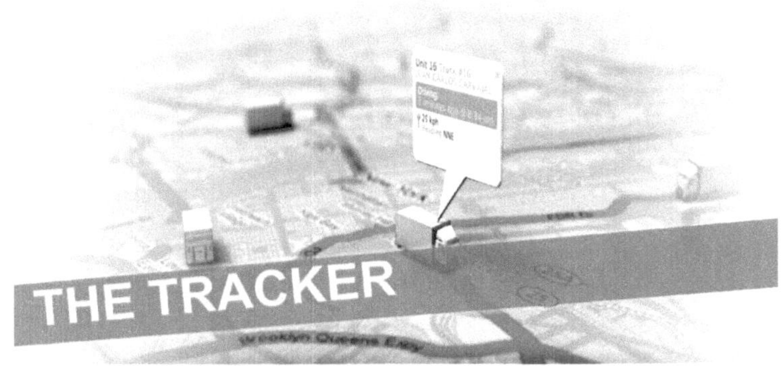

anyone that has a 100% completely hands-off automated fitness business that just brings in the cash. It's complete bullshit that consultants are teaching especially in this industry. This ultimately sets you up for failure in the long run and more work. A One Hour Trainer lifestyle fitness business can be amazing, profitable, and leveraged so you don't have to do all the heavy lifting, but don't be fooled; this is not a hands-off push this button type of business.

Here are a couple of questions for you: What parts of your business would you want to automate and systemize today as you're reading this book? How would creating better systems in your business change your business?

We want you to have a systemized workflow like an assembly line, so you can go full speed ahead without having to worry if the systems will break. This helps to create a smooth network so that you can captain the operations.

Sit back, put your seatbelt on, and let this baby fly!

Let's jump right into the five Mastery Principles that will help you design the operating systems to create that lifestyle fitness business you love.

Side note: *To be 100% clear, this chapter is not about software. It's about creating systems. Systems are made up of processes to follow in order to complete the task at hand. They can involve software for speed and efficiency, but that software needs to come along with a checklist or operating procedures to follow in order for that software to work properly. If you don't write things down step by step, you will never be able to get into the next chapter, which is leveraging your team. Your systems will crumble.*

The Tracker

In order to dominate the market, you need to show results, and the only way to show results and prove to your market and your clients that you are the best is by tracking.

If you can't measure it, you can't improve it, right?

A lot of trainers think that giving their clients a great workout is all that is needed. This industry has evolved greatly, and now, consumers are demanding more, causing fitness businesses to innovate. If you go by just delivering a great workout, you are doomed to a very difficult business that will drain you and eventually close down.

Let us talk about what to track and how to track them. We will give examples of what we use and have used in the past, but understand that these specific tracking systems may not be a fit for your business model so do your research before deciding to grab everything mentioned in this book. If you have any specific questions, head over to **www.FBMNation.com** and ask your questions inside the group so we can help you navigate these systems.

When we talk of tracking, we think of the 15 KPI's that drive a business and the results that drive customers to stay happy and loyal.

Let's talk about the 15 KPI's from Chapter 7. A majority of those KPI's can be tracked using an all-in-one CRM (Customer Relationship Management) system. These systems are great for doing all the heavy lifting for you, and with a push of a button you can track the health of your business and predict future patterns.

Before we get into specifics, let us share a quick story to put this into perspective. Having CRM systems and other trackers in place costs money, but they also give you a huge return on investment of your time, money, and stress.

We knew a trainer, Shawn, who had a business for about two years that was struggling. He had some initial success, but when we got an opportunity to look into his business, it was clear why he was having some challenges. He was too cheap to invest in tracking systems. He swore by using free Google Drive in an attempt to squeeze every penny out of profits. When we asked specific questions, he couldn't give answers or would take days to get that information.

Eventually, each month he was losing clients. We came together and installed all our Meta Burn systems. So as his client list went to zero in a couple of months, we were able to create 21 brand new clients in 30 days and eventually built it to about 42 active private clients. We took a business that went to zero and turned it into a $130,000 lifestyle fitness business all by investing in systems to track what was happening in the business.

Here are specifics on tracking the 15 KPI's:

For revenue, new sales, sessions trained, trainer performance, payroll, active clients, etc., systems that can help make tracking all of that easier and can get full reports of the health of your business with a push of a button are:

1. Mindbody

2. Zen Planner

3. Pocket Suite

4. EZ Facility

When you want to track expenses:

1. Quickbooks online

You can even go old school with tracking and use a simple spreadsheet. Don't think that you always need to pay money for a system. A tracking system can be a checklist that one of your team members follows and updates you with a report. For example, if you have a salesperson (or even if you are the main one now), they can use a simple spreadsheet called Sales/Lead Tracking that we have provided in the worksheets to go along with this book. We use this to keep things simple.

When it comes to creating systems for tracking client results, here are some software you can use, or you can take a look at the simple spreadsheets we use to track client results.

1. Vitabot – can create your own private label app with them to give clients a great customer experience plus tracking their nutrition logging from a dashboard and

tracking their weigh-ins, sleep, hydration, etc.

2. MyFitnessPal – similar to Vitabot and free, but you don't have as much control, and it's not as efficient when it comes to tracking a higher volume of people.

To track things manually as a system, there are worksheets you downloaded for the book called Client Result Tracker and Transformation Evaluation that our coaches follow and update weekly for client folders.

The Communicator

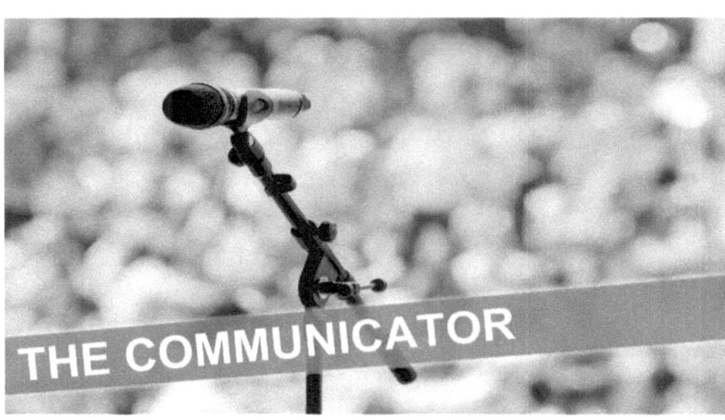

These are all systems that create communication between you and your clients or your team members. Communication systems allow you to clearly keep in touch with everyone without having to be present all the time, which helps you build that Lifestyle Fitness Business you love.

If you build a business that is based on a hope, a wish, and a prayer that your team will just take care of everything, you will be in for a rude awakening. You need to set the protocols and steps in place for communication, and you need to overlook what is being said. At the same time, clients expect to hear from you as well, so DO NOT disappear from the equation. If you want to disappear, then you need to become an investor in a business, not an owner/operator.

How are you going to get your message out to your tribe and team members?

The simplest thing to do is get a Google text line. It's free and you can track and text from your computer and from your app. You can allow team members to have access to the text line so they can reach out to clients from a centralized number, and the best part is, it's all tracked and archived. This is great because if you hand this off to an admin or your coaches, you can see how they are interacting with your clients and helps you clear up any issues when being able to refer back to past texts.

Options that cost money but have a few extra features and automation processes are:

1. Off Day Trainer – owned by our friend and colleague in the fitness industry, David Pitt

2. Skipio – they have some pretty cool features to check out

Another way to create raving fans and keep the communication as smooth as possible is opening up a free Facebook Private group. This allows you to close access off to all of Facebook and only invite in your clients so they feel comfortable sharing personal things and interacting just with their fellow tribe members. The key is to consistently post there every day, recognize clients, tag clients, and give value so there is always a 2-way flow of communication and interaction.

If you set up a group with the hopes of the clients talking to each other and you are absent or inconsistent with posting, then it will be crickets and low engagement. Even if you can't do it daily, have your admin or coaches help by contributing to the group, or appoint one or two clients as ambassadors to help.

If you are not comfortable on camera, do your best to start getting comfortable. Using Facebook Live inside of these groups allows them to connect with you on a deeper level and allows you to speak to many at once instead of one on one.

Autoresponders, which are email systems that help you build a list and communicate with a list, is crucial to have because you always want to be building a list of clients and prospects. We know open rates for emails are much lower than they used to be, but they are still money makers.

Here are a few that we have personally used:

1. Active Campaign – current system we use, mid-range price, good automation, and user-friendly.

2. Ontraport – higher end service and good automation practices but may take some time to learn

3. MailChimp – simple to use and inexpensive

4. iContact – simple to use and inexpensive

5. Infusionsoft – did not like this software at all because of price tag and complexity, but there are still a lot of businesses that use it.

The Producer

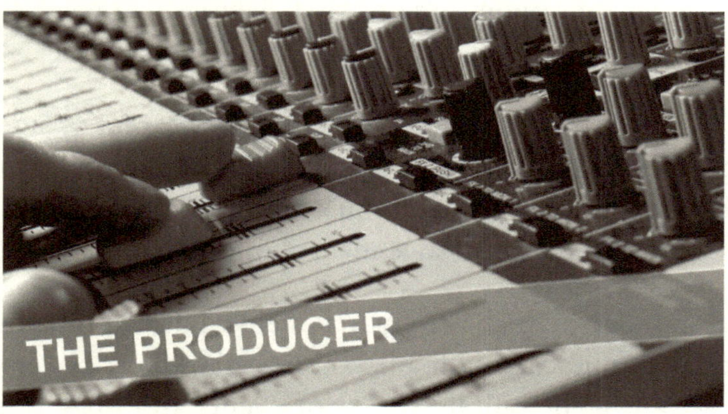

Making a movie or music needs someone in between the actors and artists and the finished product. The producer helps piece everything together, so the end product is of high value and not junk.

You need systems in place to act as a producer of great content to help create your authority within your marketplace and maintain your clients as raving fans since no one else in your market is probably putting out great content. Here's five ways you can produce great content.

First, you need to create a content calendar. This is the system that helps you organize all the content you want to put out weekly and quarterly. You never want to shoot from the hip; always have a plan of what you want to do to help make content creation faster. This is the foundation of producing. We buy a big ass calendar that hangs in our office so we can jot down content pieces, events, time-off, start and finish points of campaigns, etc. We also use what's called the Content Twister worksheet (which is in your worksheets with the book) to help us jot down a whole quarter of content and map out the main categories we want to teach, then create headlines and brief descriptions.

The first way we share content is via a weekly show we created using Facebook Live. We call it the Crush It Monday show, and it's a show all based around motivation, inspiration, and action. We try to convert those who go into Monday sluggish and turn them into avid fans who get pumped up from the show. Going live takes some time to get comfortable with, but it's a game changer. You can do this on any social media platform to be live with your audience. When your market is ready to make a decision and buy, they will remember you since you are always in their face.

If you don't feel comfortable with going live, start by using pre-recorded videos that you can share later. In your worksheets, there is the Video Flow worksheet, which gives you a simple framework of how to make video trainings with ease.

The second way to share content is via webinars. You can use either automated webinar or live webinar to share with your tribe or prospects. Automated webinars are great to use as lead magnets/free trainings to opt-in for to attract people to your business. These are great because you do the work once, and it's out there forever.

The next option is doing a live webinar. It's similar to a Facebook live, but now you can reach people who aren't just on Facebook, and you don't have to be on camera direct. You can use slides and talk over them as a live presentation. If you are camera shy, these are great to get your practice on. The main difference between live and automated is going live, you have to do the work each time you launch, but you do get to have live interaction with your market to answer questions and deepen the bond.

Webinars are great to use for exclusive trainings for your clients that only they get, which increases the value of your company to them. We use Zoom as our main software for running webinars. We have used Gotowebinar in the past, but that site can be a bit pricey.

The third way to share content is via software like Trainerize. If you want to be world class and do things your competitors aren't, this software helps you on the exercise and program design side. Whether you are an online business or offline, it works great. We shot over 300 branded video exercises with a model so we can share them with clients, create programs they can download or use on an app to follow outside the gym, or use as a lead gen to allow a prospect to try a 14-day training program for free.

This software helps you personalize workouts, or you can work from templates you pre-created to share in volume. At the same time, you can use Trainerize as an upsell to your services or even as a down sell, so if someone doesn't want to join your program just yet, you can get them on a basic virtual program to create those initial results.

Along with Trainerize, you can use Vitabot, which we discussed earlier. Trainerize is the exercise side, and Vitabot is the nutrition side where you can share recipes and meal plans.

The fourth way to share content is through spoken word. Setting up a podcast is great because sometimes people don't have time to watch a video or they just want to listen while they do other things. Podcasts are great to start with because they are simple, and you don't have to worry about staring at that "intimidating" red dot on the camera. You can go the route of ordering all these crazy pieces of hardware like expensive mics, mixer tables, different audio wires, and software to make a super high-end podcast (we have all of this and have done it this way), or you can literally buy a Shure MV51 mic, connect it to your smartphone or laptop, and start creating podcasts or audio pieces with ease.

The fifth way to share content is the written word. If you are not great at video or audio YET, you can just start with writing posts, emails, or even books like this to reach your market.

The written word allows you to slow down and collect your thoughts so that you can make everything as clear as you need. Sometimes if you are on the go and can't sit down to write, you can voice record yourself while driving, upload that to rev.com for a transcript, and edit the transcription later. This allows you to get thoughts out of your head or collect inspiration when it hits you.

The Entertainer

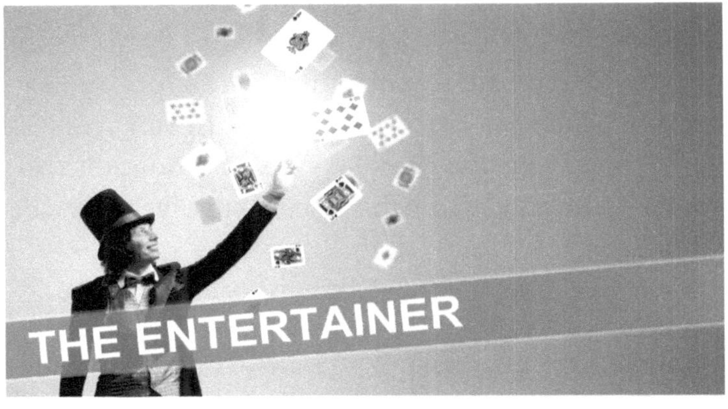

Being the producer is all about creating content systems that don't actually require you to be physically in front of your audience. That's why you need entertaining systems in place; without this, there is no personal connection. You don't want to be vanilla or hands off. You don't personally have to be the entertainer, but you have to start it so you can teach your team how you want it to run. Next is three ways to be an entertainer.

Social Events – These are made to be relaxed, fun, and inviting. Things like barbecues, races, support nights, potlucks, and even vision board events are great ways to interact with your clients on a different, more personal level. This takes you and them outside of the training and coaching environment and into the family environment. One of our most fun events was when I was Chef Rahz with my own custom apron and chef's hat, pulled out the grill, made a special drink, and served my clients a great meal.

Charity Events – These are great to get the community and your clients involved in a cause that is close to home. You can go big or small. It doesn't matter how much money you raise. It's the fact that you brought everyone together to help contribute to a cause. We did our first one back in 2009. We gathered eleven vendors and ninety people in a room for a presentation and raised over $7,000. The second charity event we did was Pushups For Charity, and we got fifteen vendors and over 150 people to participate in a push-up contest raising over $15,000 and sent a child from the Make-A-Wish foundation to Disney. Find your passion and your cause, and involve your clients to create that special bond.

Workshops – These are great for educating your clients and prospects on certain topics. You want to find a problem and solve it with your workshop. These are interactive and more professional because you are at the front of the room teaching as the leader and authority. These are great for converting prospects into clients and clients into raving fans. One event we did that crushed it was our juicing event. We had over forty people in the room, and we did a live juicing event, so they could sample different ones, learn about the benefits, buy into our philosophy, and have a chance to win a juicer. This was one of our best converting workshops.

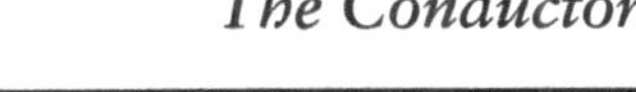

The Conductor

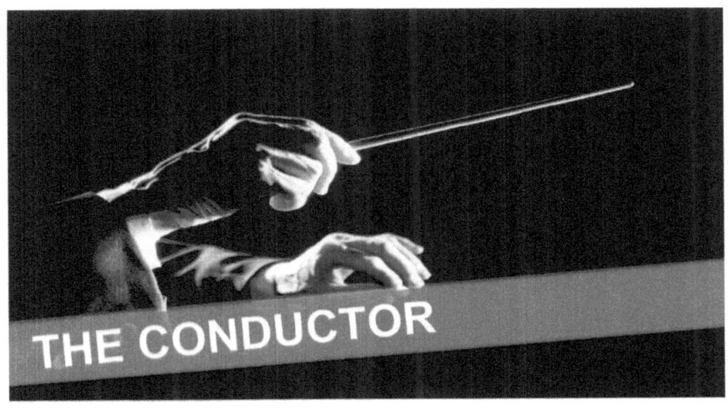

You are the conductor of all of this. People have to look at you, so you're going to keep that face on always as the leader. Strong, confident, and certain that you know where you're going. Even when at times you don't know where you're going.

But when you're the conductor, you know all the notes. You know the highs, the lows. You know exactly when you want to bring the tone down. You know when you want to lift the energy up.

What do we mean by being the conductor?

One, you want to be able to create this superhero attractive character. We have Coach Rahz, the Motivator. He's always optimistic, fired up, jacked up from the toes up and tells people what they need to hear not what they want to hear. He's the guy that helps you believe in yourself and pumps you up when you are down.

Greg, on the other hand, is Mr. Nutrition. He's an introvert, a great listener, is compassionate, and is able to walk people through step by step on making nutrition easy. He's more of the reluctant hero. Although he doesn't want to be a hero, he'll pull you across the finish line because it's in his blood to help people.

Both characters have an operating system. They have rules and ways that they act and hold themselves to the market. This does not mean that you have to be someone fake or completely different than what you currently are, but if you want to be seen as an authority or expert in your field, there are certain ways you need to hold yourself and keep other traits just for family and friends.

What is your attractive character? How do your clients view you? Post on Facebook "What is one word that describes me? I want to see how people see me." This will give you a strong indicator of how to create a character around those words.

As a conductor, you are a leader to your team. You lead from the front and need to lay out exactly what your team needs to be doing, the systems to follow, and review their performances on a quarterly basis. Just think as a conductor of an orchestra. If they allow one person to act out of line, how do you think that will affect the performance? It can destroy it. The same goes for your staff.

Your team must know that you're orchestrating every aspect of your business. We give spot checks. We show up. We send emails. We send articles that we ask them to respond to.

You want to make sure that your team sees you as a leader and sees your vision. The key to this is keeping people confident in your certainty.

As the conductor, you need systems in place for yourself. Here are some things you want in place so that business thrives and doesn't fizzle out.

1. Weekly team meetings

2. Quarterly performance reviews

3. Spot check ins with clients

4. End of week owner meetings to go over plans, numbers, and vision

5. Weekly brain-dumps

6. Weekly education for team

7. Test all your systems by overloading them to see how they handle

After reading those five mastery principles, which do you believe that you need most in your business right now?

Would it be creating tracker systems? Would it be creating more communicator systems? Would it be creating rocking production systems? Would it be creating entertaining systems so you can connect more with your tribe and prospects? Or would it be more conductor systems to create better leadership?

Any of these five would change your business in thirty to ninety days. You're going to need them all, but we want to inspire you to take one and start changing it today!

Chapter 9
LEVERAGE TEAM

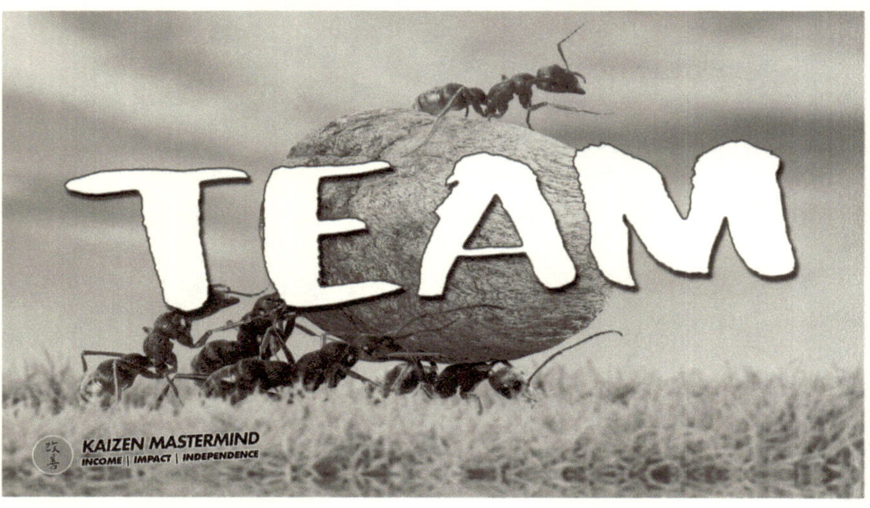

We all want a team to leverage our time and do the work we don't want to do so we can sit at home and get paid. That's the dream, right? Well, I can promise you that if you build a team, stay home, and don't overlook anything or feel like your employees will do the work you asked them to, you are in for a surprise and possibly be wiped out of business. Even with the best team in place, if you don't inspect what you expect, your team will either steal from you or not perform the necessary duties leading to unhappy customers.

This is the One Hour Trainer book. It's a concept of how to create a lifestyle fitness business so you can work on your business instead of working in it, but you still have to work. You just get to choose when, where, and control your calendar.

The biggest problem we see with trainers is they feel that they can do everything better than everyone else. Even if they want a team, they have a hard time relinquishing control and taking a step back, that whole 'soloist' mentality.

What happens with this mentality is you become overworked and stressed, you drop the ball, and you become a chief with no Indians to follow. Ultimately, it becomes a lonely journey.

When done right, a team can bring a sense of calm (most times), grade-A customer service, and a crew of soldiers ready to serve your mission. This then allows you to lead your team to victory!

With the right team in place, how big could your business grow?

We are going to teach you the five mastery principles it takes to build a world-class team.

Know Your Roles

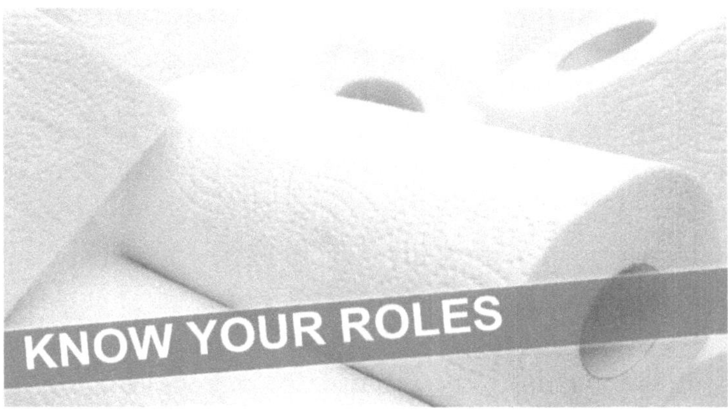

If you ever want a business that can run on its own with your visionary help, you need to clearly define the roles and responsibilities of each position. When you first start your training business, YOU become each position and wear multiple hats.

It's not fun juggling multiple tasks, especially ones you are not good at or hate doing, but it's a necessary evil to go through. It helps you understand each role, what level of skill it requires, how much you are willing to pay, and the tasks and responsibilities you can put checks and balances on.

When we first started our fitness business back in 2008, we did EVERYTHING. From training clients, setting up accounts, processing payments, tracking sessions, cleaning, video editing, video shooting, uploading files, sending out birthday cards, and so on. Your head starts to spin, wondering when this is going to stop.

This all stops once you have the chance to go through the experience at least once and then jot down exactly how that task needs to be performed. Write out every little detail of the task no matter how silly it seems. Once that's recorded, you attach that task to a position. Eventually, with every day you write something down, you will have a position fully locked up with tasks and responsibilities, and then you write out that position so you can start searching who can fill it.

We made the mistake back in the day, hiring an admin and just writing out what we were looking for and tasks tied to the position but didn't have anything written out or explained. Every day was a teaching period, and we had to explain things manually over and over. This approach can still work, but eventually, it ties you up with always teaching, the employee constantly asking questions, and when that employee leaves, you have to do it all over again.

The best approach is to write out each task in detail so if you were to hand it to someone, they would have an idea of where to start even if you weren't around. That's why we included the Job Description/Position Checklist worksheet in the packet you downloaded and printed out. This will help you create the position with tasks and the trainings required to write down. This will help you create your employee manual for each position.

Tunnel Vision

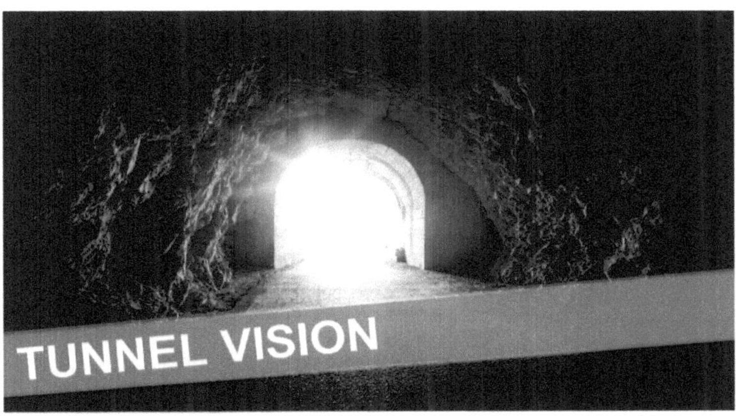

There is light at the end of the tunnel…as long as you stay the course. The moment you start doing things outside of your vision is the moment you spread yourself thin and distract yourself from the mission. We hear it often from trainers that set up their business with twenty different things they want to do and accomplish.

This becomes overwhelming and will lead to burn out very quickly. You get excited about offering a training service, then you hear how important it is to have a bootcamp in your business, then you start an online training platform so you can reach more people, then one of your clients introduces you to their workplace and you realize you have a great idea for a corporate wellness program, and if you thought it stopped there, you wanted to offer your own white label of supplements, start a nutrition program, teach kids fitness, and partner up with a massage therapist to get a different income stream.

We write this because that's exactly how our brains worked, thinking we could accomplish it all by working more hours. It took us a little over two years to dial in our focus and go down one path at a time until we figured out how to make each path work on its own.

It's not bad to dream big or want to accomplish many things, but you have to start out with one thing you want to become really good at. Once you nail that one thing, you have your team in place to leverage and open up a different path to add to your business. If you go all in all at once, both you and your team will be all over the place and you will start to become very bitter about your business.

The best thing we recommend is creating a vision board with goals and dates as well as an organization chart with built-in phases. We provided our originals that we created back in 2009 to envision our future. It wasn't the best or the most accurate with the setup, but eventually, we accomplished having the three small studios and generating $500,000 a year because we wrote it down and visualized what we wanted.

Plan a 60-minute block into your calendar this week and start writing out your grand vision, then focus on one micro vision that you want to dominate and complete by a certain date.

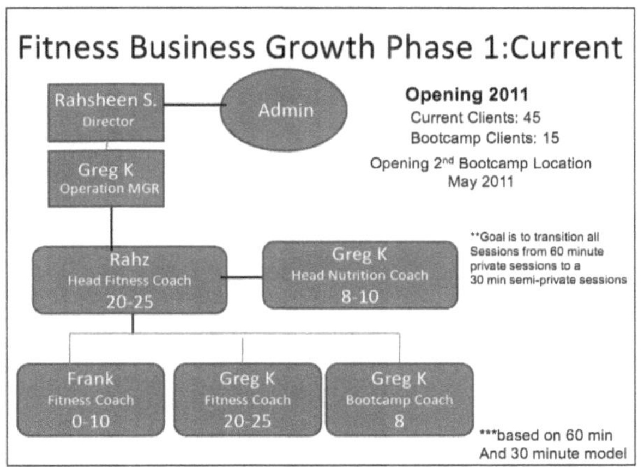
Fitness Business Growth Phase 1:Current
Rahsheen S.
Director
Admin
Greg K
Operation MGR
Rahz
Head Fitness Coach
20-25
Greg K
Head Nutrition Coach
8-10
Frank
Fitness Coach
0-10
Greg K
Fitness Coach
20-25
Greg K
Bootcamp Coach
8
Opening 2011
Current Clients: 45
Bootcamp Clients: 15
Opening 2nd Bootcamp Location
May 2011
**Goal is to transition all Sessions from 60 minute private sessions to a 30 min semi-private sessions
***based on 60 min And 30 minute model

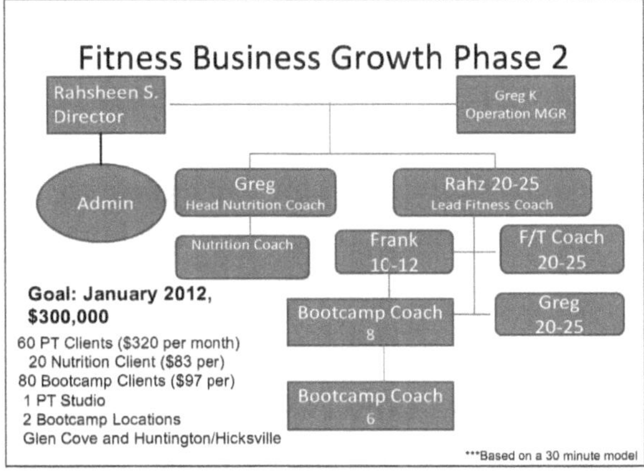
Fitness Business Growth Phase 2
Rahsheen S.
Director
Greg K
Operation MGR
Admin
Greg
Head Nutrition Coach
Rahz 20-25
Lead Fitness Coach
Nutrition Coach
Frank
10-12
F/T Coach
20-25
Bootcamp Coach
8
Greg
20-25
Bootcamp Coach
6
Goal: January 2012, $300,000
60 PT Clients ($320 per month)
20 Nutrition Client ($83 per)
80 Bootcamp Clients ($97 per)
1 PT Studio
2 Bootcamp Locations
Glen Cove and Huntington/Hicksville
***Based on a 30 minute model

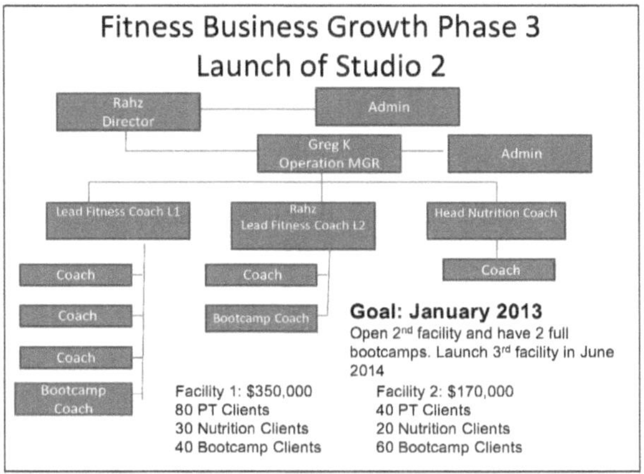
Fitness Business Growth Phase 3
Launch of Studio 2
Rahz
Director
Admin
Greg K
Operation MGR
Admin
Lead Fitness Coach L1
Rahz
Lead Fitness Coach L2
Head Nutrition Coach
Coach
Coach
Coach
Coach
Coach
Bootcamp Coach
Coach
Bootcamp Coach
Goal: January 2013
Open 2nd facility and have 2 full bootcamps. Launch 3rd facility in June 2014
Facility 1: $350,000
80 PT Clients
30 Nutrition Clients
40 Bootcamp Clients
Facility 2: $170,000
40 PT Clients
20 Nutrition Clients
60 Bootcamp Clients

Leadership Education

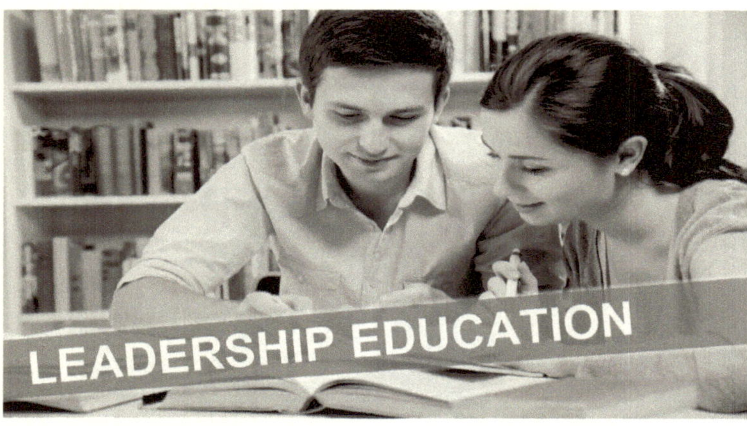

Leadership is the one thing most fitness business owners don't install. They feel that if they are the leaders, their employees should just follow. Logically it makes sense, but throughout your business, you will realize that you need more help and your people need to step up. When you expect them to step up, they don't know how and you get frustrated and mad because they aren't meeting your expectations.

The problem is you never taught them how to lead; you taught them how to follow, so how can you expect something that you never installed in the first place? There's always the fear of fitness owners that if they teach their team everything and how to be leaders that they will either leave and go on their own or will try to steal their business.

It can happen, but if you live in a scarcity mindset, you will never be able to build a leveraged business that can grow beyond what you expected. Instead, you will stay small. Whether you teach your team or not, some of them will go on their own anyway. Would you rather be large and leveraged or small and solo when that moment happens?

Educate your team each week and month about how they can

improve and start to include them in some of the creative processes. Allow them to accomplish more and be part of the overall vision. One day, you will look back and be so amazed at where your team started and where they are now.

The best place to start is to buy yourself and each team member the books *A Leader Without A Title* by Robin Sharma and *21 Irrefutable Laws Of Leadership* by John C. Maxwell as they come into your business.

Braveheart Mindset

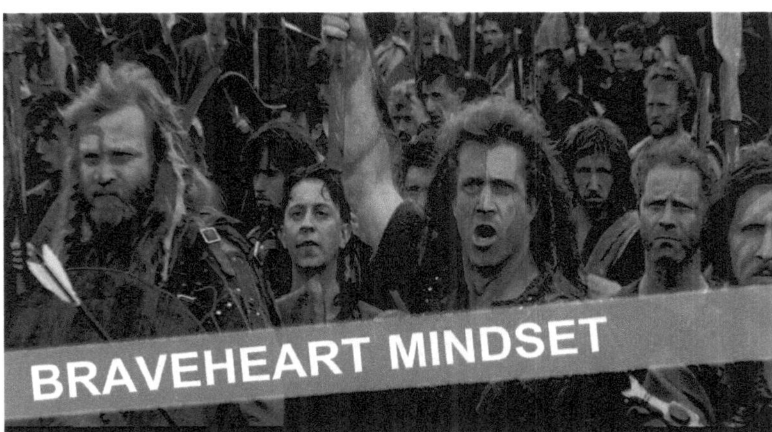

Your team is only as brave as you are. If you become the leader that sits back and expects all the work to be done, you will lose the respect and hard work of your team members. If you ever watched the movie Braveheart, William Wallace lead the Scottish army against the English. They may have lost many battles, but they ultimately won the war.

The one piece to take away from that movie is how the men were willing to fight for their freedom even though the odds were stacked against them and their lives were on the line, but they didn't get there by themselves. Many wanted to walk away, but because William had that Braveheart mindset, he led from the front and showed them what freedom was all about.

Fight from the front, and you and your team will have freedom. Fight from the back, and you will see a team of disheartened people get slaughtered. It's easy to get caught up in social media news of how you can run a successful business without doing much work and having a team around you do everything while you take home a fat check. That's the furthest thing from the truth.

The most successful leaders fight from the front and lead their team to victory. Without this mentality, even if you are solo right now, your business will never grow to where you want it to be, and eventually it will crumble.

Go watch Braveheart again!

Service above Self

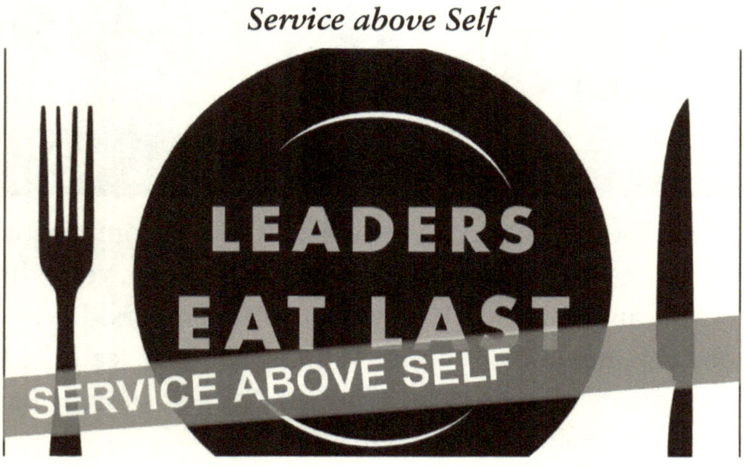

Service above self is the slogan the Rotarians live by. It's stamped on every material and each member is reminded of it often. There are times to be selfish in life, but when you learn to live by serving others over yourself, you will get everything you want.

Have you heard the quote by Zig Ziglar? "You can have everything in life you want if you will just help enough people get what they want."

It's amazing how when you start living that way, things fall into place.

That's why it's important to have monthly and quarterly performance reviews and meetings with your team and yourself. Evaluate where everyone is currently, where they want to go, and the steps in between to get there. Help your team get to where they want to go, and they will ultimately fulfill your dream of where you want to go.

It's not easy when you are working long hours, but put the service above yourself in now, and you will soon realize the One Hour Trainer lifestyle where people want to help you build your vision as long as you lead from the front and give them what they need.

Chapter 10
FLIGHT PLAN

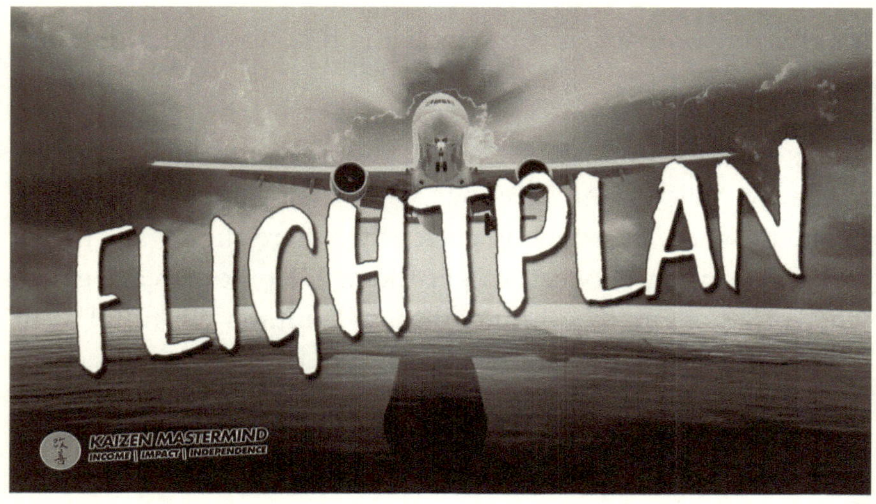

"If you fail to plan, you plan to fail" – Ben Franklin

Seminars, books, and coaches that don't give you a plan only set you up to fail. The fact of the matter is that if you're going to be successful in creating a lifestyle fitness business, you're going to require a plan that's going to give you specific details of what tasks and projects there are and when they need to be completed in order for you to arrive at a specific outcome. That is what this chapter is all about.

You've had the opportunity to go through nine different chapters and hear many success stories of why you need to be focused on building a lifestyle fitness business, so that you can have a profitable business that you love so that you can avoid being burnt out, bitter and broke. **During this chapter, we are going to detail a specific 90-day roadmap** that's going to give you three specific projects and the actions required in order for you to take off to the next level.

Why is a roadmap necessary, you ask?

It's very simple. Most personal trainers fail due to the fact that they have a lack of clarity. They are not clear about the direction they want their business to head or the overall vision. If you lack clarity, any shiny object is going to distract you and deflect you from what you need to be focused on.

This can cause them to shoot from the hip. If you don't know what you want, then you try different things each week wondering why nothing is working. They wake up in a state of confusion and frustration because they don't have a focus.

From that frustration and confusion comes busy work—moving papers around, browsing the internet, posting on Facebook, or sitting inside your gym hoping the phone will ring. If you got into business to make an impact and make more income, then why aren't you doing income-producing activities every day? Your lifestyle fitness business soon will become a lifestyle of no business.

When you decide to make daily plans, focus on three major projects each quarter, and take action each day; you will become the One Hour Trainer, the trainer that actually has a life, money, and opportunity to do what they want, when they want, and with whom they want to do it with.

Every day, you need to be focused on creating marketing to attract your ideal client, converting those prospects into leads and leads into customers, and delivering a world-class service that your clients will tell everyone in their circle about.

I want to share with you a case study of one of our amazing mastermind attendees who came to a two-day mastermind, and was blown away by the systems, the strategies, and the tools that we employ to our Kaizen Mastermind clients each and every month so that they can grow and scale a profitable fitness business that creates a lifestyle for themselves. He was able to take a few of those skill sets and strategies that we shared with him over two days and immediately created an impact on his business by installing those systems in his business.

Nicholas Vidal, PA

Plant Strength

www.PlantStrength.com

I came to Fitness Business Intensive back in October 2017 for a 2-Day mastermind event with Rahz and Greg. What a great experience and environment to focus on building your business and taking it to the next level. They over delivered and helped me gain clarity on my business and shift my focus to content creation and lead generation.

Before the event, I was struggling with clarity on my message, my ideal client, and programming, and I had a big problem with lead generation. I was sort of stuck. This event was very intimate and intense. This wasn't a hyped-up seminar where you leave with nothing set in place. I actually left with a 90-day Flight Plan specifically for my business.

My biggest problem in the past was information overload. I get too much information at one time and don't know where to start.

The event helped me to build my authority in the Gut Health market, understanding how to utilize other FB groups to build credibility with my content, and filling out the 90-Day Flight Plan really helped take my business to the next level. I now have complete focus on my mission at hand.

Just within seven days of completing the mastermind, I signed up two new clients to my online program for a total of $2,400 in new revenue. I want to thank Rahz and Greg for helping me map out my flight plan and for all the great connections I made at the mastermind.

Nick's 90-Day Flight Plan

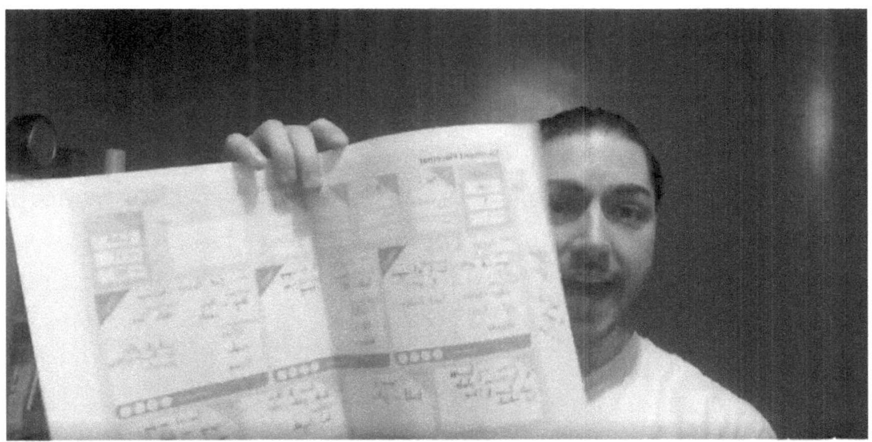

We want to share with you the five mastery principles for creating a 90-day roadmap to land this plane.

Plan it

The first principle is you have to plan it. You must plan specifically for what are the key things you need to do in order to move forward. This is called a braindump. We want you to take out a sheet of paper, set an alarm clock for thirty minutes, and unload everything you have in your mind about how you want to grow your business, how you want to attract your ideal client, and what projects, what marketing campaigns, and systems you need to put in place. Put it all out on paper. That's the first step.

Prioritize it

The next step is you need to prioritize it. How do you prioritize it? This is where you're going to get organized. So now you're going to set three different chunks: activities that are about attracting/marketing, activities that are about converting/sales, and activities that are about delivery/systems. Each of your projects can be broken down into one of those three chunks; that's the organization factor, what we call prioritize it.

Post it

The third step where you're going to post it. Open up your 90-day roadmap, and chunk it down into three specific projects that you're going to do over the next ninety days; we want to eliminate any of the shiny object's syndrome, all of the things that distract you from moving forward.

Publish it

The fourth step is to publish it. You're going to set deadlines for each of those three projects. And this deadline has to be really, really tight because you don't want to give yourself an out.

Produce it

The last step is to produce it. Do the work. Action, action, action. See, you can plan it, you can prioritize it, you can post it, and you can publish it, but if you don't produce it, you are just spinning your wheels without getting paid. The only thing we get paid for is completing things, so if you don't get these projects completed, then you'll never attract your clients, convert those clients, deliver the service, or build a lifestyle fitness business that you love.

Those are the five mastery principles for creating a rock solid 90-day roadmap to success. That's it. Done! The book is over!

You don't think we would just end it on you like that, right? Anti-climactic and still leaves you wondering, "What the hell do I do?" The reason we made this chapter much smaller is because we wanted you to grasp the simplicity of the principles, but now we want to show you how you really do this with a detailed training on how to fill out the Flight Plan worksheet found at **www.TheOneHourTrainer.com/worksheets**. It's much easier to follow along with us in a training then it is to read it in the book. We want this book to have a major impact on your business; that's why there are multiple trainings and worksheets to go along with this book.

Before you fill in your 90-Day Roadmap, we want to thank you from the bottom of our hearts for picking up this book and investing in yourself. It takes hard work to build a lifestyle fitness business, but it's well worth it when you follow the ten chapters in this book.

You are going to hit roadblocks and question whether or not if you can still do this. Trust us; we have been through hell numerous times, but we never gave up, and now we have a business that works for us instead of us working for it. It's normal to go through the pits in order to reach the path of success.

If you want to burst right through those roadblocks so you can achieve the success you are after and avoid the mistakes we made building our business that almost shut us down and could use some help along the way, then I have a special gift for you.

If you do this 90-Day Roadmap, go to our Facebook page at **www.FBMNation.com**, and post a picture of your roadmap, we are going to gift you a complimentary 30-minute roadmap audit. We'll go over your roadmap with you, and the cool part about it is that we'll make sure that all three projects are properly aligned with your vision, your theme, and the actions needed in order to accomplish them. This is not a sales call. This is simply because you took the action. You did the work. You read the book. You supported us. We want to support you and your success.

From myself, Greg, the entire Kaizen Mastermind, and all of the personal trainers and coaches that have inspired and motivated us to create this book so that you can grow and create a lifestyle fitness business, thank you for reading, and God bless.

Discover How The Kaizen Mastermind Can Transform Your Business Into An Asset That Works For You, Makes You Money, And Gives You Freedom.

Apply For A Position At The Round Table At
www.KaizenMembers.com

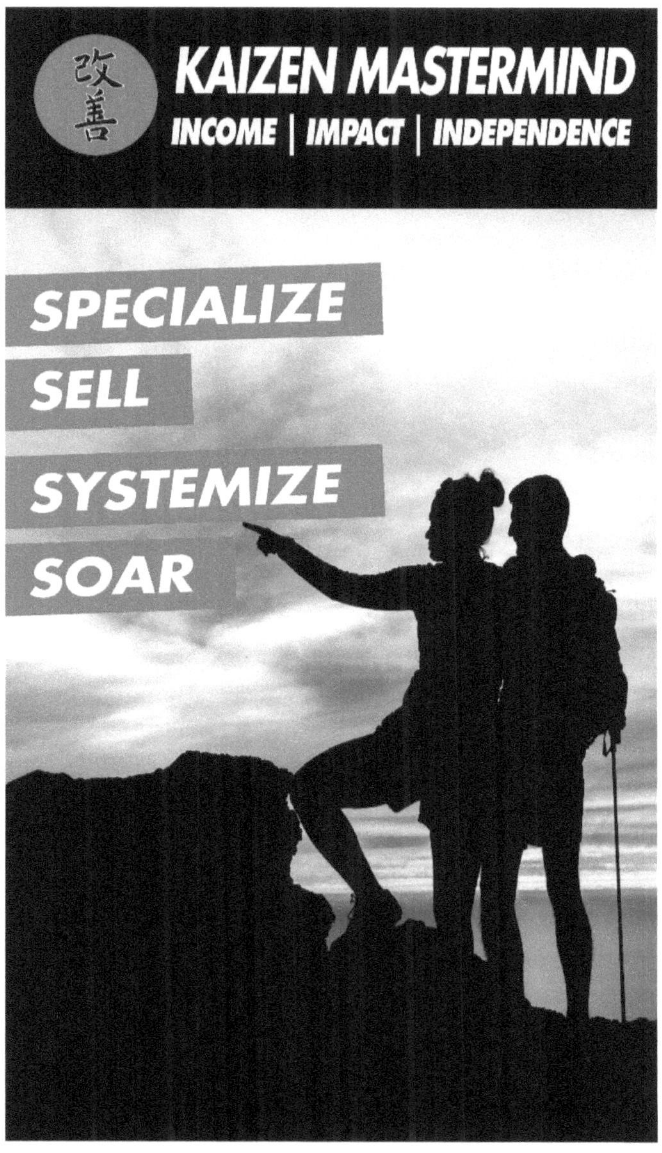